Roger Brown

Against My Better Judgment: An Intimate Memoir of an Eminent Gay Psychologist

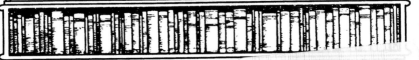

D1019212

The book is fascinating for the human questions it raises–not just about Roger Brown, not just about gay men, but about the human condition that we face as we approach the later seasons of life and career. Why, in the first place, does Roger Brown need to tell this story, a story that is always indecorous, sometimes tawdry? Is he reliving, almost in the form of theater, the root conflict of his long marriage to his lover–a conflict between tender intimacy and raw sexuality? Is it a tale of internalizing the departed lover he grieves: Roger now becoming the 'cruiser' that Al had been, but still searching for tenderness in the three young lovers whom he takes on one after the other in this quest? I say 'theater,' for Roger Brown has always had an attachment to and knowledge of the forms of theater–whether in drama or opera–that made 'all life a stage' for him in more than a metaphoric sense. Or, one cannot help but ask, is the book a delayed expression of the chagrin that distinguished gay men must feel, once emerged from the closet–the expression of a need to tell straight friends after the fact but right in the eye 'what it's really like'? In fact, one senses in the telling, despite all differences between the straight and the gay, that it may not be all that different. Most marriages are strained by tensions (many not unlike the one recounted here), the death of a partner often releases an unrequited sexuality in the survivor, and grief is sometimes relieved by a fevered and painful quest for new partners. And, lest we slight theater, Shakespeare's *King Lear* reminds us that the sufferings of our waning powers often generate searing new insights, that in time and with turmoil, lead us to 'see with our ears.'

Against My Better Judgement is a moving, disturbing, and immensely human book. It speaks to Roger Brown's greatness and courage as a human being. We are all in his debt for his having dared to write it, and for his having succeeded so vividly in doing so."

Jerome Bruner, PhD
Research Professor of Psychology,
New York University

"**R**oger Brown has written a searing personal memoir that will leave no reader unmoved. Brown, a distinguished psychologist at Harvard University, member of the National Academy of Sciences, and author of several acclaimed textbooks and enduring studies of the psychological aspects of language, is also now a lonely, desperate man, bereaved at the death of his homosexual partner of over 40 years.

He tells a shockingly straightforward story of his response to his grief; of his loneliness; of his stumbling attempts to find love and acceptance and peace in the arms of homosexual prostitutes; and of his tortured self-loathing after his attempts to love are not returned. Told in graceful prose, the story mixes the tragic with the comic and absurd in such a way that produces art.

This book addresses the specifically human occasion of widowerhood, whether homosexual or heterosexual. It forthrightly recounts what may happen when the ties of long years of companionship are broken. It depicts the problems in trying desperately and compulsively to establish intimacy and in experiencing unrequited love. It is an affecting human document that takes the reader, perhaps unwillingly, because it is often an 'in your face' unpretty story, beyond the shock of unrecognition of this renowned, erudite, and cultured psychologist, to the understanding of the universal and complex nature of human attachments.

Professor Brown, in his self-exposure, may have written his most penetrating psychological study in his depiction of the human condition in late life. One must wonder, with Freud, '. . . why a man has to be (so depressed) before he can be accessible to a truth of this kind.'"

Philip S. Holzman, PhD
Esther and Sidney R. Rabb
Professor of Psychology, Emeritus,
Harvard University

Harrington Park Press
An Imprint of The Haworth Press, Inc.

Against My Better Judgment

An Intimate Memoir of an Eminent Gay Psychologist

HAWORTH Gay & Lesbian Studies
John P. De Cecco, PhD
Editor in Chief

Against My Better Judgment

An Intimate Memoir of an Eminent Gay Psychologist

Roger Brown

Harrington Park Press
An Imprint of The Haworth Press, Inc.
New York • London

Published by

Harrington Park Press, an imprint of The Haworth Press, Inc., 10 Alice Street, Binghamton, NY 13904-1580

Cover photo by Richard Scudder.

Cover designed by Marylouise E. Doyle.

Library of Congress Cataloging-in-Publication Data

Brown, Roger, 1925-
   Against my better judgment : an intimate memoir of an eminent gay psychologist / Roger Brown.
      p.   cm.
   ISBN 1-56023-888-7 (alk. paper).
   1. Brown, Roger, 1925-   . 2. Gay men–Biography. 3. Aged gay men–Social conditions.
4. Homosexuality, Male. I. Title.
HQ75.8.B76A3   1996
306.76'62'092–dc20   96-25488
                                                                                           CIP

This book is dedicated with love
to Albert, Bob, and Jim

ABOUT THE AUTHOR

Roger Brown, PhD, was the John Lindsley Professor of Psychology at Harvard University. His doctorate is from the University of Michigan (1952), and he taught at Harvard for 40 years either social psychology or psycholinguistics. A member of the American Academy of Arts and Sciences and of the National Academy of Sciences, he was awarded the international prize of the Fondation Fyssen in Paris in 1985. In 1992 Roger Brown received the *Phi Beta Kappa* prize for excellence in teaching. On February 1, 1994, Roger Brown became Professor, *Emeritus.* Asked why he wrote the present book, he said, "It's a contribution to the anthropologic record."

CONTENTS

Acknowledgments

Because I have always been a very private person, I always knew that this intimate and honest book would shock many dear friends–at least at first. It was never my purpose to shock but only to be very truthful. However, if I kept steadily in mind, as I wrote, a sense of being shocking, it would interfere with telling the truth. That problem was there from the start because I do not know how to type and I love my secretary, Mrs. Sarah Goldstron, who has typed many books for me over a period of twenty-five years and I did not want to worry about Sarah's reaction to every sentence I wrote. So I went outside Harvard to Bette James and asked her and her associate to do the clerical work. Dear Bette has been wonderful in not overtly reacting to anything and so, as you will see, leaving me completely unrestrained. She has also been wonderful in other ways, especially in her willingness to put in extra time and speed things up when that was what I needed. In not asking Sarah Goldston to type the manuscript I probably did Sarah an injustice. She has shown herself fully capable of adapting to my unconventional lifestyle, yet I did not want to risk a friendship so central to my life. So I thank Bette James and Sarah Goldston together for their great work and great friendship.

I have been very ambivalent about this book from the start, repeatedly asking myself, "Why am I writing this? It can only damage my reputation." And so I am especially grateful to a few friends who stiffened my backbone. Dr. Jim Groves, Dr. Gregg Solomon, Dr. Randolph Catlin, and Mr. Philip Leon are four of the smartest people I know and the fact that they all "got it" and "liked it" made an enormous difference from the very start. Later, Dr. Ellen Langer and Nancy Hemenway were not only supportive but made excellent suggestions. After the book was finished and in production, I rather dreaded its actual appearance, yet the comments on the manuscript by Jerome Bruner and Philip Holzman, two great psychologists whom I have always admired, were themselves reward enough for the whole enterprise.

Albert's beloved sister Mollie encouraged me to write this book, even though it contains disclosures about her brother which she might have preferred to leave private. I believe she showed the courage and openness of her brother and I am grateful to her.

To my family and my friends who know me only in my guarded conventional life, I apologize for the shock and hope it will not cost me their affection.

Finally, what can I say to Albert and to my three guys: Skip, Grant, and Patrick? Thank you for letting me love you and thank you for loving me back.

Introduction

There are some gaps in gay literature that I expect to fill with this memoir.

A memoir is true, true of the author. Autobiographical, but not so complete as an autobiography, a memoir is free to concentrate on a particular period and subject. This one mainly concentrates on five years, my sixty-fifth until my seventieth (1989-1994), and the subject is love and sex. The combination of subject and age define one gap the work is intended to fill. In a time when the public is expected to hear the story of every sort of stigmatized person and, hearing, to understand, why should "dirty old men" alone be excluded? Why even those who are queer as well as dirty? Mind you, we are not asking to be liked. In a good light I can barely like myself.

Reading gay novels (and I have read all those one can possibly get through), you find that all the heroes are young, usually under thirty. You would think there were no gay writers over forty. And of course, that is very nearly true. AIDS has killed off the literary flower of a whole generation. Still there are in fact quite a few sexagenarians and septuagenarians around. They have not died of AIDS because for them the great era of sex fun that preceded AIDS, the 1960s and 1970s, was a window of no opportunity. They were already too old to fuck or be fucked. I offer myself as their spokesman.

Gay men in their later years do occasionally appear in gay fiction. Usually they are represented with some cruelty, perhaps as a group of envious onlookers at some function for young men, sucking on their breath mints and sucking in their guts. The lack of sympathy is quite astonishing in works that cheerfully accept every sort of sexual indulgence. The gay community comes across in fiction as a community of the young, good-looking, potent, and well-hung. Probably the author is unable to identify with any other type and expects his readers to feel the same way. But the function of art is, as George Eliot says in *Middlemarch*, "to widen our sympathies, amplify experience and extend our contact with our fellow men beyond our personal life."

Old gay men in stable same-sex unions are not very different from old men in straight unions—unless they lose a spouse. Then the difference is great. The elderly widower is a social prize who can be introduced to a different prospective bride every evening if he so chooses—and many do. Not infrequently he will have picked out a potential successor from among his wife's friends before her demise. For me the case proved quite otherwise, and so it does, I think, for most gay widowers.

I have wondered, sometimes with envy and sometimes not, why I was different, why I became such a loose cannon sexually and romantically, so unlike my straight friends and also so unlike the married gay man I had been for forty years. The essential answer lay not with being gay but with being "unanchored," though these two conditions are highly correlated.

Children are marvelous anchors and so are close relatives who live nearby; they hold you in place, in chocks, even stocks. I had neither children nor nearby relatives but only an adoptive family of men and women gathered over many years, in part for their unconditionally supportive ways. I felt no restriction from this quarter or any other.

But I was lonely. "Lots of people are lonely. What's so special about you?" This small challenge came from Edwige, my housekeeper, in the days before she met her friend Andrew.

"Nothing that makes me deserving of sympathy," I hastily responded, hoping to win a little. "I think and behave so crazily because I have had too much spare cash and time and have seen too many Italian operas."

Loneliness is not the same as the lack of a strong sexual-romantic bond, but the two are close. For everyone, the category of persons who might meet this need is very specific and usually small. For me, the category was large enough but disastrously out of reach: handsome young men with a touch of vulnerability about them.

Vulnerability is easy to find, but the young and handsome seemed ruled out for me at sixty-six and beyond because of the ageism of gay men. I was pretty sure of this because I myself felt it so strongly. Albert Gilman and I were young together and passionate together and so were able to love one another–in changing ways, to be sure–over many years; but when I thought of making a new beginning, the idea of doing so with someone my own age was distasteful. And so I had to suppose that young gay men felt that way about me. I was categorically eliminated as an object of attraction to anyone for whom I felt an attraction. There could be no point at all in going to bars or running a "personals" ad. Imagine how it would read: "Cultivated man of 66 seeks 20-year-old for summer fun." No, no point at all; and so it would have been Alice-sit-by-the-Fire were it not for the blessed institution of male prostitution.

Women, straight or lesbian, cannot grasp the ageism of gay men. I have often been told by Al's sister Mollie and by kind women friends that from many points of view I was something of a catch and there must surely be young or youngish men who would feel the same. There are. But being a "catch" or finding a companion does not solve the problem of loneliness. Loneliness is a problem of the heart. The question is: Are there any achievements, possessions, or qualities of character that can cause a man in his twenties to fall in love with a man in his sixties? I thought probably not, but for several years it was more interesting and more exigent to try to find out than to do anything else.

I made three trials, and that is what this book is mostly about. The trials fill another gap in gay literature. What happens when an old man with a very advanced education becomes sexually and romantically involved with a young man of little education? I can answer that one for you now. The old man, especially if he is a psychologist, discovers that his idea of human nature has been formed by a cohort of very like-minded folks with certain values, knowledge, and qualities of character. Going outside that cohort in a deep way, one discovers how far from universal truth his notions of humanity have been.

This is not an autobiography in any usual sense. There are no tiresome forebears, no dysfunctional family or agonized "coming of age." In fact, there is no family at all, but just enough background to establish the discontinuity, the incongruity of the last years. Because incongruity is the truth about human nature.

In personality, it seems to me, anything goes. Not in the moral sense. Not in the sense that every sort of action is morally acceptable, but in the descriptive sense that any combination of traits or actions that can be imagined can be found. How we contrive still to be surprised at, to find newsworthy, the fact that the corrupt politician, the serial killer, the child abuser—next door—is described by all his neighbors as "the nicest guy you'd ever hope to meet." How we do that, I do not know. But there is something that makes "evaluative consistency" everyman's theory of personality.

Chapter 1

Prelude to the Afternoon of a Faun

One day in the fall semester of 1951, Albert Gilman said to me: "I want you to read these abstracts especially carefully because one of the authors is in my department and I don't want to be embarrassed by clumsy writing."

We were both graduate students supported by the G.I. Bill of Rights, at the University of Michigan; Albert was in English and I was in psychology. In 1951 we had been together for the unusually long period of four years. In 1989 we were still together, making our total time as a couple forty years, which must be some kind of record.

As a graduate student at Michigan and for several years afterward, Albert wrote abstracts of articles for the *Shakespeare Quarterly.* He did this pedestrian task because he did almost no other publishing and felt it was a duty as well as something to put down in the annual report to the Dean. Asking me to have a critical look at a set of abstracts on this day in 1951 was no rare event. In fact, once we had lived together long enough to establish individual responsibilities, Albert asked me to read over everything that would be made public—even course descriptions for catalogs. He believed me to be an unusually graceful writer–graceful at least for a psychologist.

Albert did not do scholarly publishing of a more prestigious sort because he believed himself to be ham-fisted, almost crippled as a writer of English. He had no trouble writing comments, some as long as essays, on student papers, but any assignment to write something his colleagues would read terrified him. All his academic life he dodged assignments and offices that entailed writing. His colleagues never understood, because Albert was a superb committee member and speaker, and they kept trying to elect him to positions he would decline to fill.

I agreed with Albert that his writing was pretty bad, not as bad as he thought, but it was labored and redundant, with never a happy phrase, literally never. I tried to conceal from Albert this hurtful evaluation, but he knew, and he probably thought I had trouble respecting someone who wrote as he did—but speaking is not writing. In writing you have to supply the full context—in words—and that makes writing a skill unevenly distributed in the population. When you speak the context is there—the setting, the listener, the shared past. Albert's speaking over meals, at parties, in class was witty, subtle, unpredictable, and that is the way his friends, and the thousands of students he eventually had, thought of him.

The request to read something often created a tense situation. While I was generally very willing to do the job and concerned to guard Albert's self-esteem, if he asked when I was concentrating on my own work or felt pressured for time, there would be irritation in my voice, and Albert almost always heard it. At best it was a humiliating situation for him—he, the English major, asking help in writing English from me, a non-English major. I remember that his dear tobacco-stained hands trembled a little whenever he had to ask.

"I can't find anything wrong with this one. It's fine just as it is."

"That means you can't be bothered. What about the logic of the conclusion? Does it follow from the way I've put the premises?"

Just to be done with it, almost arbitrarily, I moved around a few words.

"There, you see, it's completely different. And the whole thing has taken you exactly seventeen minutes. This is one thing you can do for me, anyway."

I did not ask what the things were I could not do because I had a feeling he might have a long list, and that giving sexual satisfaction might be on it.

* * *

How did Al and I meet? We cruised one another in a men's room; that's what young scholars in small towns did in those days. It was a very routine thing; but times change, and eventually we rather enjoyed answering "How did you two meet?" because, to young gay men, it seemed sordid and unpromising.

"What's it like to live with the same person for forty years?" asked young Barry, a student of Albert's.

"You just turn around and it's forty years," Al answered.

One time Al asked me: "Which of us would you rather died first?"

"Oh, pray to God it will be me." It wasn't. Al died of lung cancer in 1989.

I expected the devastation that followed. What I did not expect came after the eventual abatement of pain–after about eighteen months–a regression to adolescence when the exigent need had been to find someone to love, a Primary Other, to glue me to life. So exigent that, at the hopeless age of sixty-six and after a prostate operation that left me usually impotent, I found I must work at fulfilling this need and found ways of doing so, ways that were humiliating sometimes and romantically thrilling at other times. Why the need for a Primary Other should be so urgent is too deep a question for me, but there is no doubt that it is for almost everyone.

Nothing had prepared me for the sex and romance of later life. Not Freud, not psychology as a whole, not what I knew of world literature. Only Thomas Mann's *Death in Venice* and Vladimir Nabokov's *Lolita* even come to mind, and both Aschenbach and Humbert Humbert were decades younger than I.

If sex and romance were a surprise to me in my sixties, and they were, there was a greater surprise: the relationship called "male prostitution," which the world thinks of as purely manipulative, need not be. It can be, of course. It can be fleeting and unfeeling, but it can also become richly human, long-lasting, compassionate, and not recognizably sexual at all. It took three young men and five years to teach me that.

The great thing about my forty-year marriage, I came to think, was not the happiness it brought, but the freedom to lay away the search for an ideal love and work on something more manageable and satisfying; for me: psycholinguistics or the psychology of language. The marriage gave Albert the opportunity to live much of his life with Shakespeare–an improvement on the endless mulling over of his relationship to me.

There are many ways to cruise a men's room, and Albert and I knew them all, but there is only one that eases the student's anxiety at totally taking time off. You must bring a book and, sitting on the pot, door closed, read with as much concentration as is possible in a duck blind. When your duck arrives and settles his feathers in an adjoining booth, you abandon your text and concentrate on the foot and ankle visible to you. A certain amount of shifting or foot tapping is meaningless neurological overflow. What you want to be on the lookout for is PATTERN. There are several kinds of interpretable patterns, but the easiest to read is the foot that moves consistently in your direction; first the toe, then the heel, always by very small increments, never enough to justify a challenge or even to be seen by any but the devoted cryptanalyst. The nightmare possibility is a deep voice saying: "Hey bo, what's up?"

The most dispiriting sight in these circumstances is a polished black oxford with black silk hose over a hairless blue-veined ankle. Even one such can empty half a dozen stalls. The fact that the foot and ankle are the first exposed "parts,"—the bait—as it were, seems to have had far-reaching consequences for men's fashions. Even academic deans find themselves wearing white athletic socks and Reeboks, though they certainly know not why.

Back in the stalls, one's own foot should move in the manner of the chap next door, edging in his direction. There is in the end an inescapable Rubicon. One or the other must risk . . . CONTACT. Actually, it is not a great risk; unless there is a clearly voluntary companionate pressure, anything less can be erased with an apology. However, once pressure is assayed and returned, the scene becomes electric with erotic potential.

Some will drop to their knees; some, even more incautious, will look under and up. There are, after all, additional essential, inspections to be made, but once a mutuality of desire is established, things happen very fast. If someone's standards are not met, the whole interaction can end with overdone flushings and slam-bang exits. If both parties are agreeable, the possibilities are diverse and exciting, the excitement intensified by the possibility that aliens, wanting only a restroom, will blunder upon the horrifying scene.

Do not think that this kind of "tearoom" cruising was peculiar to the University of Michigan or to Albert and me. Eventually all the universities in the Big Ten took off all the doors in all the men's rooms, and even this extreme denial of privacy was not fully effective.

In any university, it was not all the men's rooms that served as meeting places, but just a few; you had to know which. The surest sign was a "glory hole," a glans-sized hole in the wall between stalls. Sometimes these looked as if they had been smoothly drilled, and one wondered who did such drilling, and when. Desperate universities sometimes put steel plates over popular glory holes, and that gave the impression of an attempt to control wild beasts, determined to get at one another. Some bathrooms served as "tearooms" for many years and in that respect were like certain public buildings in Washington and Dublin that have been starling roosts for a century or more.

Universities also had men's rooms in which people urinated, moved their bowels, and washed their hands, but there was almost no overlap between these and "tearooms." The very idea is disgusting, but of course the fixtures were the same, since tearooms were never intended to be what they became. The slightly comical result is that white porcelain is, as some pornography directors know, a sexual turn-on for just that age group most interested in pornography.

Albert and I were satisfied with what we saw of one another, and Albert, ever the leader, stepped out of the stall into the room with his pants around his knees. "Come on out," he whispered.

"Someone might come in."

"They won't. This building is empty after six."

"If anyone does, I'm gonna run for it."

At 6'3" I was a good five inches taller than Al, but he was strong, and he bent me back and planted a wet kiss on my mouth. Too wet to suit me.

"Open your mouth!" I did, and Al's tongue was inside, hungrily darting. "Lizard-like," I thought squeamishly. I was very excited but at the same time would have liked to draw the back of my hand over my mouth to dry it a bit. This wasn't dentistry, after all.

"Damn it! Kiss right! Use your tongue!"

I tried but didn't do very well—clearly not carried away. So Al shifted to my cock, cherry red and so rigid it quivered. He swallowed it whole and it filled his mouth but did not choke him.

"Fuck my mouth! Go in and out!"

After a time Al straightened up calmly and said, as if he were inviting me to lick an ice cream cone: "Try mine." I did and noticed the head was almost purple and there was a little nick in the ruff, as if someone had been so carried away as to try a bite. I slipped a hand to his firm white butt, found the tender spot, and tested its tension as if it were a trampoline.

"Oh yeah, I like that. Put your finger in a little way. I wish I could take it but I can't. I've never been able to."

Then Al reached behind me and, with no preparation, thrust in two dry fingers as far as they would go. I shuddered and my mouth opened all the way, releasing a great flow of saliva.

"That's right. That's good. That's what you like." Al added a third finger and, paying no attention to my "ouches" and "ows," went vigorously and mechanically to work. Both splurged on one another and we laughed as we zipped up our flies.

"That was hot. Do you want to get together again?"

"Definitely."

"My name is Albert—Al."

"I'm Roger."

"Okay, Roger, here's my number. Call anytime you want to meet. Don't worry about my roommates, Reed and Bill. They're both queer and can be trusted to take messages. We live in a big single room, second floor. On State Street. Near the movie."

"One thing before you leave." I took Al in my arms and kissed him tenderly. He looked absolutely amazed.

It was a good thing Al and I met as we did, in a swirl of lust and flesh, because it was going to be a while. You see, I fell in love, first love, if you don't count my mother, and love promptly turned off lust, but lust or desire there would have to be.

I knew vaguely of Freud's theory of the black Madonna and the white Madonna (Venus and Elizabeth in Wagner's *Tannhäuser*) and had read that some men had trouble conflating the two and became impotent when they attempted to have a serious love; I supposed that was now my problem with Albert. Alone, I could create a fantasy and become easily potent, but with my Elizabeth, my most improbable Elizabeth, I was hopelessly limp.

Al was surprisingly patient: "You're a beautiful man and have not had anything like my experience. It will work out and I can wait." It did work out, and when it did it was like the confluence of the mighty waters of the Mississippi and the Amazon. Of course there is no such confluence in geography, but if there were it would be a big effect, and so it was when Venus and Elizabeth became one.

Once it happens, the problem is forever solved; it is as if a dam has been swept away. I went a little crazy and talked about Albert and the wonders of love to all sorts of people, even straight people, even girlfriends, and when Al and I could get in the same room and lock the door we stripped down and sucked and penetrated everything anatomy permits. And it was not enough. It was never enough.

Reed, one of the roommates, finding the door unlocked one day, glanced in and quickly jumped back. "It looked like the Rape of the Sabines," he said afterwards, with Roger so deeply tanned and much taller and Albert breadbox white as he always is and on the bottom for once.

One day Al, looking puckish, quoted *Twelfth Night* with the change of one word:

> Some are born great
> Some achieve greatness
> Some have greatness thrust into 'em.

Albert meant by this that it seemed to him that the most natural way for the two of us to have sex was for him to do the fucking. For just a moment I thought he was making a claim to have the larger penis, and I would have contested that, since we were about the same size, but then I realized that he was just talking about what was mutually comfortable. And that became the "default" posture, always possible to change under special inspiration but as a routine maximally pleasurable.

"I never said I would give up cruising, you know. It's not really the sex that's important. It's the excitement. The danger and the chase."

I had never thought of raising the question of fidelity because I could not imagine that there would be any temptation. What we had together was incomparably better than anything a stranger could offer. It engaged the whole of the body and spirit. It was a transcendent experience, the best thing in life. Apparently not, though. Al wanted anonymous sex as well.

Incredulous, I eventually went back to one men's room to see what could motivate Albert's desecration. It was ugly and smelly and impersonal, a place for taking a dump. But when a pair of white socks and sturdy tanned legs appeared next door and commenced the courtship waltz, I grew curious about the man above and excited myself with possible images. What ensued was not transcendent, but it was exciting, and while the excitement lasted I did not care about anything else. It wiped out the rest of the world, including Albert. With consummation everything snapped back into place, assuming usual values and the preceding madness was just a little mess to clean up. Casual sex belittles love, because it seems that a biochemical state and an object adequately stimulating can totally overcome the most particular passion. That is what makes casual sex intolerable to a person in love.

But with Albert I learned that toleration of casual cruising was the cost of an enduring bond. For years we played a game of "catch-up." He led the way, having the greater appetite and know-how. When he got too far ahead I dropped my books and my pants and did a little catching up. The score was never even, but probably there was a rather stable interval between us. It was fair enough, because Al had no interest in love with his partners; he was a little like the female praying mantis which bites off the head of her partner after breeding, whereas I was more interested in the other person and disposed to fantasy about lovers other than Albert and, in that way, less "faithful" than he. I spread my romantic thoughts over a small population and he engaged a larger population but with no romance at all. It was an awkward harnessing that moved by fits and starts but did move in the sense that it permitted both of us to take degrees and then teaching positions and spend most of our time as scholars. We were also good companions, both interested in theater, opera, and music. We eventually amassed an amount of shared experience that made us irreplaceable as companions for one another.

* * *

In 1949 I met a girl, Marian Sanders, and fell in love. Not with Marian, but with the idea of being in love with a girl. Marian was a graduate student in the English Department with Al. She was very pretty, funny, and responsive. Al liked her better than any other student in the department and wanted me to meet her. We went together to a student production of *The Importance of Being Earnest.*

You may remember that the play opens in the London flat of Algernon Moncrieff:

> *Algernon:* "Did you hear what I was playing, Lane?"
> *Lane:* "I didn't think it polite to listen, sir."

In all the audience only Marian and I laughed. For the moment I did not know why I had laughed, but I was enchanted that Marian had also laughed—only Marian. It might mean that we had both taken in what Oscar Wilde intended, which was not at all obvious. For a good part of Act I, I thought about the first two lines and what was funny about them. The answer was quite psycholinguistic. *Hear* and *listen* are almost synonymous, but not quite. Hearing is involuntary; if you are not deaf and a sound is within range and loud enough, you hear it. It's none of your doing and you do not necessarily pay attention.

Listening is voluntary. You can't listen to something unless you can hear it, of course, but listening goes beyond hearing in that it does necessarily involve attention. Why should Lane, a servingman, not think it polite to listen to Algy's playing, which he could not help hearing? Well, because, at a minimum, paying attention verges on eavesdropping; it could be an imposition, an embarrassment. Something an impeccable servingman like Lane would not do.

The hear-listen contrast, I realized, is not the only one of its kind in English. There are also see-look at and smell-sniff contrasting on an involuntary-voluntary axis.

In the next few lines of the play, Algy asks Lane to make a judgment of his playing, which is something that attentive listening would make possible but mere hearing need not. Lane is quite wise to disclaim listening since he might have got the judgment wrong:

> *Algernon:* I'm sorry for that for your sake. I don't play accurately—anyone can play accurately—but I play with wonderful expression. As far as the piano is concerned sentiment is my forte. I keep science for life.

Again Marian and I laughed and we continued to laugh at every speech. In the intermission after Act I, I asked Marian why Lane's line "I didn't think it polite to listen, sir" was a funny line.

"I'm not sure, but there is something absurd about its being impolite to listen when Algy's playing loud enough to be heard."

"I think that's right," I said, delighted with so apt an answer, and I went on to expand upon it as I have done here.

Marian looked at me, worship in her eyes. "That's wonderful. Psycholinguistics explains how the line accomplishes its effect, though Wilde certainly had no knowledge of psycholinguistics."

"He had his brilliant linguistic intuition—and you have it too."

In Act III we had even more fun with a line of Lady Bracknell's:

> Her unhappy father is, I am glad to say, under the impression that she is attending a more than usually lengthy lecture by the University Extension Scheme on the Influence of a Permanent Income on Thought.

This convulsed both of us. "Can't you see members of the House of Lords sitting in easy chairs—dozing? That's the influence of a permanent income on thought."

"No," said Marian. "Tenured full professors of English asleep in the faculty club. You know what I'd love to do on April Fool's Day? Put up colloquium announcements all around the department with that title and as speaker 'Lady Augusta Bracknell.' I bet nobody'd get it. They'd just troop in dutifully to hear one more obscure lecture."

A real meeting of minds, it was, for both of us. I thought I was in love and Marian, in fact, was. She lived with her sister Joan, who was in anthropology, much quieter than Marian but with the same sense of humor. Al liked her a lot because she was modest and understanding and very bright. We four became steady double dates all the time we were in Michigan, but Al and I were the lovers. We did not even kiss the girls or put our arms around them. This strange relationship was possible because the girls were serious Roman Catholics. They did not push their faith and were not offended when we made jokes about nuns and saints, but they kept steadfastly to their faith: mass every Sunday morning, very serious about every Christian duty, and, most conveniently for us, convinced that Christian ladies never discussed sex and never took the lead with men. They were dear girls who loved us and were wonderfully happy with us and somehow thought it would go on forever.

Marian had had a boyfriend before me—just one—and so she had some knowledge that there was a pleasant physical side possible. She would hold my arm sometimes when we walked in the street and just once tried for my hand at the movies. But since I jumped as if these things violated the incest taboo, she gave up.

Once Marian confided to me that she and her "ex" used to go to drive-in movies and neck and that she had just loved it. I did not take the hint.

Now I must confide here what I did not confide to her. There are creatures from outer space living among you, more different from you than you can imagine. We come out of pods at night and assume human bodies. You cannot distinguish us. We look just like you. The difference is in our perceptions—of the female sex. Where you see tits and ass and legs and I have no idea what else, we see faces above and below are skirts to the ground. Underneath the skirts, what? Pillars of sugar and spice, for all we know.

Don't tell me I have only to open my eyes at the beach to see voluptuous breasts and round little behinds. We just don't see them. And we also cannot imagine the functions or activities of the lower part of the female form; none at all, we would guess. To be sure, they are always going off by themselves to "ladies' rooms"—Marian and Joan would often do this twice on a date—but what goes on there, if anything, is no business of ours.

Psychologists like to point out that one or another animal species lives in a different perceptual world from the human world—seeing no colors, perhaps, or hearing higher frequencies than we can. No need to look to another species; differences fully as great distinguish the queer human from the straight human. That is why I perfectly understand what straight men mean when they say they can't imagine what one man sees in another. Of course they can't. You have to come from outer space.

Marian did not realize how hopeless it was to wish for physical intimacy, but she thought it unladylike to press and also counterproductive, since it might endanger what we had—the intimacy of likeminded friends. It probably did not occur to her that Albert and I might be homosexual lovers, since there weren't any on TV or in the movies, and we never gave any sign in public.

Later on, when the foursome broke up, friends told Marian and Joan that *of course* Albert and Roger were homosexual. Whether they believed it then, or ever, only they know. They must have, many years later, when they lived in San Francisco and Albert and I, still living together after forty years, came out from Boston to see them once a year. My guess is that both early and late they knew as much as they wanted to know. We were from the start and always the most important men in their lives, and they were too wise to spoil the love we all felt and the happy times we had together by dwelling on something in which they had no part to play.

Marian once said: "When you're with us in San Francisco, I feel I can't stand it that you will leave in a few days, but I know that you don't want to see that." And once when we talked, with inconsiderate enthusiasm, about various friends back in Boston, Joan, who was usually very private about her feelings, said: "We like to think we're special to you." Once or twice Al and I went with them to spend Christmas day with their nephew's family and all the relatives. These modern Californians surely figured out the basic story of Albert and Roger, the boyfriends at a great distance of Aunt Marian and Aunt Joan, but I am certain that the sisters never tolerated any speculation in their presence about our sex lives.

Marian and Joan are not absurd figures. They are strong and kind and original. In 1991 in San Francisco I had occasion to bring them together for dinner with a one-time graduate student of mine, Tom Moore; and beforehand, I did a lot of explaining about Marian and Joan to Tom, since, although he was young, he was "cool," and I thought he needed to know what to expect. Everybody laughed a lot at dinner and Tom confided to me: "They're wonderful."

Marian and Joan's mother had died even before we met them as students, but they had a living father, who mostly traveled, but visited them once a year or less. When he dropped by, they showered him with love, but he kept his independence: "I may see you for breakfast at the League tomorrow, but I may not be there. If I'm not, just go ahead without me."

In his eighties, the old chap got seriously sick and had no choice but to come live with his daughters. And how happy they were to have him to look after. They even ensconced him in the apartment's only bedroom and moved themselves to a sofa and a daybed. After several years of loving care, he died. The girls kept his bedroom as he had left it as a kind of shrine and, because they could not bear to part with his old car, they had it put on blocks in storage where it could be visited.

As students in Ann Arbor we all did have a happy time. Escorting the women to parties or plays or just to the seven o'clock or nine o'clock showings at the State Theater gave the men a feeling of normality which they enjoyed. And the girls were fun.

Normality reached its apogee and very nearly tumbled me into a life of deception and sexual frustration on a certain Sunday when my parents drove up to Ann Arbor and had dinner with Albert and me. The girls were also there but I made the meal, since I was still in a "new bride" phase, showing how well I could cook. The day went very well in that Marian and my mother liked one another a lot; I was pleased by that, and in a serene mood of familial closeness I thought: "Why can't it be like this? There's no real reason Marian and I can't get married. Sex is clearly not very important to her and our fun together is. I could still break away from the hopeless relation with Albert and the debased business of homosexual cruising and live happily with my colleagues and students and family in the bosom of heterosexuality."

After dinner, since everyone seemed to want to be quiet, I put on a recording of the Beethoven violin concerto at the slow movement. I was in the right mood and this sublime music choked me with emotion. At this point Marian, who was sitting with her feet up and her eyes closed, said: "God, that music is *so* depressing."

Ah, Marian, dear, that remark cost you a husband. But you are better off without *this* husband. That was the last time I considered marriage and going straight. I was better off too. Forty years later Marian and I were still friends, because we still had fun together and she tried hard to share my musical enthusiasms. However, at a performance of *Rosenkavalier* I turned to meet her eyes during the Act III trio, to share the wonderful moment, and caught her sneaking a nap. Thank you, God, for sparing me forty years of such moments and sparing Marian too. Late in life I played Marian's role and tried to share the musical enthusiasms of three young men, one at a time, not to deceive them but to be close, and it was no fun. Disco and country and western are not for me.

* * *

It was a Friday afternoon in November, gray and drizzly, the kind of day that makes you wonder if you really care to live through the weekend. I was guiltily putting a few things in the plastic overnight bag my mother had obtained with green stamps from her grocery shopping.

"I don't see why you have to go home to see your mother every weekend. If you stayed we could do something. I never knew anyone who went home every weekend."

"I know; I feel bad about it. I've tried to explain—my mother and I have an unhealthy crazy close relationship. She's very dependent on me. She tells me I give her the only happiness she has. And until I met you I felt the same way. It's incredible, but each time we part we both have to choke back tears. We are both always thinking of the fact that one day before long we will be parting forever."

"Does she tell you you must come every weekend?"

"No, I just see the happiness I give her and the preparations she has made—she makes all my favorite dishes. I started out wrong, going every weekend because at first I really felt like it, and was homesick here. Now she expects it and looks forward to it, and if I break the pattern now she will really be hurt and I'll feel guilty."

"And what about me? I'm not sitting in this apartment all weekend. You're giving in to your compulsion to go home, and that gives me the right to give in to my compulsion to cruise."

"Do you think I enjoy going home? There's nothing to do there except look at the damn television. I think about you all the time."

"That may be, but it's not enough. When you go home, I go out. That's the way it's going to be."

"You go out anyway, during the week when I'm home."

"Yes, but I try to control it, and I never go out if we have something to do together. One of the reasons I went into this relationship in the first place was to break the cruising habit. It was beginning to control my life, taking all my spare time, keeping me from forming any real friendships. I was very happy that you broke that up. Remember the first dinner party we went to? I told you this was the way I had always wanted to live."

"Yes, and I felt wonderful about that. At first, anyway. I thought it meant you were through with cruising because what we had together was so much better. But it turns out you still cruise, only not as much, but I have to live with the thought that that is probably what you would rather be doing. It spoils things for me. I want to love wholeheartedly, not half-assedly."

"You want to love wholeheartedly and yet you will not stay here one weekend."

"Even if I stayed, I would feel that you were discontent. Years of casual sex have spoiled you as a lover. You are great at having sex—with me and probably anyone—but in between there is no expressed affection. You never touch me except when we are having sex. You never meet my eyes or say something loving. It's embarrassing even to talk about it with you because you are so far out of it."

"It's not because of casual sex; it's just the way I am. I know I'm not good at expressing affection. None of the men in my family are. Their wives all complain about it."

"Well, never mind, my dear. I miss it and think I really need it, but I realize that on a deeper level you are completely reliable. You never have failed me in anything important. Why don't I go home this weekend and tell my family I will not be able to come next weekend and try to break the pattern gently. Why don't you call Marian and Joan and invite them to take in a movie? I'll be back in time for supper on Sunday. Is that okay?"

Then, with a wicked little smile, Albert said, "Don't tell me you're leaving without kissing?" and he turned up his cheek to invite a routine smack. He did that always from then on whenever we parted, and if I forgot he acted horrified and said something like "Where's your great love today?" It came across as mild mockery.

When I got home I found I could not tell my parents I wouldn't be coming next week.

* * *

In 1951 I finished my dissertation, which was on authoritarianism and personality rigidity. Authoritarianism, assessed with a paper-and-pencil instrument called the "F Scale," was the most popular topic in social psychology in the 1950s. After World War II, American fear of Soviet expansionism led to the Cold War between the North Atlantic Treaty Organization and the eastern Warsaw Pact nations. In the United States, a paranoid fear of internal Communism was common. In 1953, with the election of a Republican Congress, Senator Joseph McCarthy became chairman of the Senate Permanent Investigations Subcommittee, with results that are well known. Many American social psychologists did not feel the extreme fear of internal Communism, called the "Cold War mentality," and for us the book called *The Authoritarian Personality* (Adorno, Frenkel-Brunswik, Levinson, and Sanford), published in 1950, became a rallying point for both research and politics.

The F Scale which was developed in *The Authoritarian Personality* was also called a scale of "Potentiality for Fascism," and the book stigmatized not the Communist Left but the neo-Fascist Right. Most of the research done with the F Scale showed authoritarians to be a bad lot: sexually repressed, ethnocentric, antagonistic to minorities (including homosexuals), stupid, and conventional. I have always thought that most work in political psychology, including my own dissertation, was in part a way of striking back through research at the Cold War mentality and McCarthyism.

A social psychologist at Michigan State, Milton Rokeach, had discovered that high scorers on the F Scale (authoritarians) tended to be so rigid in problem solving that, having found one sort of solution that regularly worked with arithmetic problems of a certain type, they failed to notice when a shorter, simpler kind of solution became possible, even though it was made clear to them that the simpler solution was preferred. The problems used (known as the water bottle problems in psychological research) ask subjects how they could measure out various quantities of water using bottles of specified sizes. Each bottle can only measure its full volume and so no gradations are marked. The best solution is the shortest solution. The experimenter (in this case Dr. Rokeach) begins by demonstrating the solution of one problem such as the following:

Given   Capacity containers: thirty-one quarts, sixty-one quarts, and four quarts

Obtain   Twenty-two quarts

Solution   Fill the bottle that holds sixty-one quarts, from it fill the thirty-one quart bottle; from the remainder withdraw four quarts twice. In short: sixty-one minus thirty-one minus four two times equals twenty-two.

The first six problems can all be solved by the same method which may be abstractly characterized as: largest minus second-largest minus smallest, two times. These first problems established a kind of intellectual "set" and subjects usually see that there is one formula that handles all problems and are pleased to have found it. Beginning with the seventh problem, however, while the previously used formula continues to work, a simpler solution also becomes available. For example:

Given   Forty-nine, twenty-three, and three
Obtain   Twenty
Solution   Forty-nine minus twenty-three minus three two times
           equals twenty or, alternatively and preferably: twenty-
           three minus three equals twenty.

The effect of the set is very strong. Many subjects continue using the original formula and never do notice the shorter and superior alternative. Rokeach used the water problems as an index of general mental rigidity with the rigidity score being the number of problems presented before the subject found the shorter solution. What he discovered was that children who scored high on the F Scale (the more authoritarian children) were more rigid on the water bottle problems than children who scored low on the F Scale (non-authoritarians). The same contrast appeared with college students. This neat result was consistent with a rather large literature showing that authoritarianism was associated with cognitive rigidity.

Some of us at the University of Michigan were very taken with Rokeach's demonstration and, for several years, we attempted to replicate the finding with the students enrolled in the psychology laboratory courses. However, we never succeeded; that is, we never found that rigidity for the water bottle problems was significantly related to authoritarianism as measured by the F Scale. I was so puzzled by the difference between Rokeach's findings and the results in our laboratory that I made an exceptionally fine-grained analysis of the methods used in the two laboratories, even going so far as to sit in on one of Rokeach's sessions. What I discovered was a large but not-deliberate difference in the social atmosphere prevailing when the experiment was conducted in the different laboratories.

Rokeach had his subjects write their answers in blue books and in general created a serious, test-taking, ego-involving situation. The teaching fellows in our laboratory were very casual young people who gave the impression that they were conducting a demonstration of no great importance. It seemed likely to me that in a formal test-taking situation, authoritarians would feel sufficiently threatened to "freeze" onto a solution that worked and fail to notice shorter alternatives when these became available. In a relaxed, more playful situation, I thought authoritarians might perform as flexibly as non-authoritarians.

What I did for my doctoral research was deliberately test the hypothesis that contrasting atmospheres produced contrasting results. Instead of letting the Rokeach-style setting vary by accident from the style in our laboratory, I produced the atmosphere difference deliberately by writing scripts and picking actors to administer the tests. It worked, but rather weakly.

The idea was a good one. In general form, it was that *what* a given test or procedure measured–what aspect of personality was tapped–could be influenced by the social atmosphere in which it was administered. But the effect was not strong, and even under extreme torture by statistics only a barely significant result appeared. I was actually repelled–by my thesis, and from the study of personality. The experimental study of personality suggested to me a topic infinitely sensitive–the atmosphere did after all have a satisfying effect–and, at the same time, was extremely unsatisfying. The effect was so small I was not sure it was real. I confess that I like larger effects that I am sure I understand.

The graduate student society asked me to report on the work in a colloquium. That colloquium had a big effect on my life. Someone put up, all around the department, announcements that included a sketch of me giving the talk. The sketch knocked me out. A tall figure was inevitable, since I was six feet three inches tall. But the figure was very masculine, broad shouldered, large boned, and affable, actually smiling. It had never occurred to me that anyone could see me that way. The image was not what I got from my mirror. To be sure, Marian seemed to see me that way, but I always thought Marian was under suspicion of wanting to please. Albert told me I was handsome, but that did not carry much weight, since I was clearly not handsome *enough* to make him into the kind of lover I wanted him to be.

My usual self-image was perhaps some years out of date, a skinny adolescent with minor acne. And since I was homosexual and always had been, I assumed that it showed as it did in some of my friends; therefore I must look effeminate. And sour of face, I supposed, since I was alienated from my society. The sketch suggested this was all wrong, or at least that I could be seen otherwise. No one told me it was a poor likeness; several people told me it was excellent. The Navy, in which I had served for three years, while failing to make a man of the inner me had, apparently, given me the look of a man. I held this look firmly in my head for at least twenty years.

The colloquium itself taught me that bad research, or inconclusive if you like, did not necessarily mean a bad story. I should have known that because Michigan let me teach many independent lecture courses while still a graduate student. My courses went well: "History and Systems," "Sensation and Perception," "Psychology of Language," "Psychological Laboratory" and, in the extension service, "Theories of Personality." I had made good stories out of many bad experiments.

* * *

Albert and I bought Marian and Joan a Victor Red Seal record called "Golden Duets," on which one could hear such Golden Age opera stars as Caruso and Antonio Scotti, Giovanni Martinelli and Rosa Ponselle, Tito Schipa and Lucrezia Bori. We all loved that record and played it again and again. The title "Golden Duets" signified forever the Ann Arbor years, when we ourselves were a couple of Golden Duets. Especially, I think, for Joan, who would ask, even forty years later, "Remember 'Golden Duet's?" We all knew her nostalgia was for certain years and not just the record.

"Golden Duets" was playing one night when Al threw a bombshell: "Roger has accepted the Harvard offer."

What duet was playing? I can't recall, but it should have been "Un de felice" from *La Traviata,* in which Violetta, who has been offered love by Alfredo, bids him to be off because she can offer no more than friendship.

Joan's response to Al's announcement was: "Congratulations, Roger. That's a great honor."

Marian gasped as if she had been punched in the stomach. Collecting herself, she said to me: "If you go to Harvard, I'm going into a nunnery, that's all." This was extreme enough and absurd enough to pass as a joke requiring no serious answer, but it was more than a joke. Marian was a devout Catholic and had gone to a high school where she was taught by nuns. She looked back on those years as happy and uncomplicated. She knew what living in a nunnery was like and might therefore intend to be understood literally. Except that one could not quite believe in Sister Marian; there was too much irreverent fun just beneath the piety.

What Marian expected me to get from her startling pronouncement was the extremity and exclusiveness of her attachment to one man. If he were unattainable, she would have none. I was put in Hamlet's position, as if by moving to Harvard I were saying to her: "Get thee to a nunnery."

Joan recognized that Marian's pronouncement was also directed at her. "You wouldn't really, would you?"

For Joan it was a threat of desertion; she had pretty much given up on a degree in Anthropology. Joan was actually very dependent on her more assertive sister. If Marian were to go into a nunnery, there was some question whether Joan alone could manage. Roger would be gone, and Albert was bound to leave in another year or so; and if Marian were also to go, what would happen to Joan? For Joan there was a kind of implicit threat in what Marian said.

Albert continued: "He doesn't have to go to Harvard. Michigan has matched their offer, so he could stay right here."

"Oh, well, then do it. What's so great about Harvard? I'm sure Michigan is just as good, and in psychology it's the best, isn't it?" Shamelessly Marian added: "Think how hard it will be on your folks, especially your mother, if you go away when you don't have to."

I had of course thought of my parents and already knew how hard it would be. My mother certainly wanted me to stay at Michigan but her wish to dissuade me was reined in by her sense of parental obligation: "Couldn't you be just as happy at Michigan?"

"I think it might be good for me to go somewhere else. After all, I've been at Michigan since I was a freshman, taken all three degrees there, and studied with just about every member of the department. But I won't go unless you agree to spend half the academic year in Cambridge. It would be good for you. You need a change as much as I do and there's really nothing to hold you here in the winter. I'm sure I could find you a nice little apartment near me."

"What about Puddy? We couldn't leave her." Puddy was a pussy cat adopted in the days of the canary in the animated cartoon who said, "I t'ought I 'taw a puddy 'tat. I did. I 'taw a puddy cat," and then bashed the cat with a mallet or equivalent.

"Puddy could come too. We'd get a cage and put her in the back seat." In fact, we did eventually do that, but along the way Puddy of course had to "go." Many times. Once she escaped me, darted out the door, and skittered around on the icy steppes of Ontario. I remember my poor father crunching around in the snow, plaintively calling: "Pud-dee! Pud-dee!" It makes a very poor name for a dignified man to call aloud.

Without committing themselves to spend time in Cambridge, my parents voiced no objection to my moving there. It was not my parents and not Marian and Joan and not the reputations of Harvard and Michigan that made me decide on Harvard; it was the state of things between me and Albert, which was something no one else at all ever heard about.

* * *

As far as behavior was concerned, Al and I followed the fairly stable catch-up pattern I have described, but my inner life was in a perpetual stew. I wanted wholehearted romantic love as it appears in the operas of Puccini, if nowhere else. I wanted to be held, caressed, doted on, and spoken to with endearments. Sometimes I felt positively swollen with love for Albert, but if I put my arm on his shoulder he would shake it off and say "People can see," or if I tried to hold his hand he would snatch it away and say "What's the matter with you?" If I made an explicit complaint he would do what I asked, usually overdo it, so as to mock the feeling behind it. This left me feeling needy and perpetually ruminating over whether I should stay with Albert or try to find someone who would be more responsive.

In fact, I made several efforts to leave him, all of them, I think, at bedtime. "Do you know you were gone six hours this afternoon and evening? What on earth were you doing all that time?"

"I told you I was going cruising."

"For six hours? How is that possible?"

Al just shrugged.

"You must have been with someone you are interested in."

"How often do I have to tell you I'm not interested in meeting someone? I spent the time reading *Coriolanus* for tomorrow's class and watching for some 'action' which never materialized. It was very boring."

"I don't believe you. No one can spend six hours cruising. You're meeting someone. I've suspected it for some time."

"Here we go again. It's paranoia time. Must we go through this routine?"

"I'm not paranoid, and this time it's not routine. I'm going to spend the night at the Union and tomorrow I'm moving out." I began to collect toilet articles and a change of clothing, but I was so mad I could not think just what I would need. "You really are a bastard! Leaving me to spend the day alone. It doesn't matter if you were only cruising! What kind of a degenerate can cruise for six hours?"

"You were absorbed in your work when I went out and enjoying it. You love analyzing data and writing. I can't get that kind of pleasure from my work. I can't sit here all day just reading."

"I don't care! I've had it." And I slammed out and over to check in at the Union. In the little room they gave me I started to undress and noticed that I had left behind the papers I was grading. Also my comb and toothbrush. I thought about tomorrow and how hard it would be to find an apartment and move. Especially now, in exam time. And I had wasted most of the day fretting over what Al was doing. Probably he was doing just what he said and having a very depressing time. The poor guy did not have much fun. He enjoyed the classroom and larking around with students, but most things in academic life bored him. I phoned home.

"It occurs to me that you had some Shakespeare abstracts you wanted me to look over today. I'd better come back and do that."

"I wish you would; they're overdue. After you finish we might call the girls and ask them if they want to meet us for a beer at the Pretzel Bell."

I was as glad to get home as if I had been away for a week. At bedtime Al came in my room for the ritual kiss and had the gall to say: "By the way, I've decided to forgive you." He went to his room and fell asleep in five minutes. I tossed and turned for two hours, thinking I probably should not have come back. How I resented this physiological advantage of his; he could always go promptly to sleep.

A woman who once said I looked needy went on to say: "And Al does too." Albert needy? How could he be, with the cornucopia of love I poured over his head? Could it be that it was not the kind of love he needed and may even have detracted from what was needed? If cruising brought what was needed, then romance was not the answer. Say rather all-out physical abandon and imagination, roughness and impersonality. From pornographic movies seen late in life I have learned that I was not totally abandoned and so not very "hot." There were things I would not do, postures I would not strike. I would not put my feet over my shoulders and I set limits on depth of penetration. Pain and dignity and, I thought, safety defined the boundaries. I can remember asking him: "Are you sure this is safe?" and his answer: "If it isn't, then an awful lot of people are in trouble."

I wasn't tough either and would not pretend. Nor rough, nor dominant, nor impersonal. In short, not what he most liked, I suspect. Therefore he was also needy.

I hated myself for losing every trial of separation from Albert by being the first to cry "Hold! Enough," and this is the reason I accepted the Harvard offer. Acceptance was irreversible and it would put me at a distance. When I told Albert my decision, his chief concern seemed to be his own work: "I have a full year of writing to do and I was counting on your help."

"You will be fine by yourself and Marian will be happy to go over everything and act as editor. She's an excellent writer, you know."

Locked into leaving by my decision, I proceeded in the summer of 1951 to take back my decision by working on the prospect of getting back together. Al was to finish his thesis and find a position at one of the universities in Boston. Al went along with my talk and mostly agreed with it because he had no wish to leave me. He did not expect to fall in love with someone else. The very idea of falling in love was a joke to him, something out of operetta. I seemed to him nice-looking and smart, a man with a future and so an excellent long-term partner. Sexual satisfaction was not, as everyone knew, to be found in marriage. If I would realize that and stop worrying about what he was doing, I would be fine.

While I talked about the separation as temporary, as something to be undone as soon as possible, in my heart I hoped for one of two outcomes I did not discuss. The departure might end my attachment to Albert. At Harvard I might find a rich and wonderful world that would enable me to ditch him. Or by actually leaving I might put an irresistible pressure on Al and "bring him to heel," as it were—as the sexually constant lifetime companion I thought I wanted.

Albert was aware of the treacherous hopes that lay beneath my talk. It may have seemed likely that the year's separation would accomplish emotional detachment, especially when I was appointed resident tutor in one of the Harvard houses and given a suite of rooms and free meals in return for meeting once a week with small groups of unimaginably glamorous young men. But Albert did not worry. He knew that, in spite of Harvard's diversions, I was stuck on him forever and would spend a lot of time pining for him and writing more letters than he really wanted to answer.

So I left Ann Arbor. Albert did write his thesis, with Marian happily helping, and then he got an assistant professorship at Boston University and the poor chap was entangled with me for life. Marian gave up work on her doctorate and took preliminary steps in the direction of a nunnery, but then Joan had a nervous breakdown and Marian had to give up the nunnery and take charge of their lives. Al and I lost contact with them for five years.

* * *

In my first year at Harvard I was given two daunting teaching assignments: "Psychology of Language" for the Psychology Department, because George Miller, whose course it was, had resigned and gone five miles up the Charles River to MIT; and "Introduction to Social Psychology" for the Department of Social Relations, because Gardner Lindzey, who had made the course very popular, had bigger fish to fry.

For the language course I assigned George Miller's textbook *Language and Communication* but taught *around* it rather than *from* it; and so it happened that when I published my own textbook in 1958 (*Words and Things*) there was no topical overlap with Miller's book. He was attracted by topics that made some use of mathematics, especially communication theory. I thought *his* topics should be studied by reading *his* book—but myself preferred to work up all the more verbal, more speculative topics such as metaphor, phonetic symbolism, language and thought, and the acquisition of language. E.G. Boring, who was "Mr. Psychology" in those days, when I told him how I had worked, described the books in *Contemporary Psychology*, a journal of reviews of which he was the first editor, as a "patrix-matrix" pair.

When Professor Gordon Allport told me that I was to teach social psychology, I protested: "I'm not a social psychologist; I'm an experimental psychologist. I've only had one introductory half-course in social psych."

"You're a social psychologist now," said Professor Allport, who was an eminent, slightly epicene man in a dark blue suit with a vest.

The first time I taught the course it was all stimulus-response learning theory, very much in the style of John Dollard and Neal Miller, who were learning theorists at Yale, and I never did get to anything more social than imitation. Students would scratch their heads and say: "There must be more to social psychology than this." "No," I would assure them, "that's all there is."

I might have said more exactly, "That's all I know that is at all relevant," and that was because stimulus-response learning theory had been the number one, intellectually complex subject at Michigan. It was the principal interest of the chairman, Donald Marquis, and it was the subject that attracted the sharpest graduate students. It was preeminent very much as cognition is today.

I taught social psychology every year for twelve years, first at Harvard and then at MIT, and the expectations of the students led me to explore in many directions for content that would satisfy them and me. When I published my own first text in that field, there was no stimulus-response psychology in it at all, but rather a unique amalgamation of language, conformity, intelligence, moral reasoning, mass phenomena, and so on, which turned out to be sensationally popular with teachers and students and was adopted by almost every leading university in the English-speaking world. It stayed in print without revision for more than twenty years.

My research affiliation at Harvard was with Jerome Bruner's Cognition Project. The Project was doing experiments on category (or concept) formation using the theoretical language of attributes and criteriality. I asked Bruner to read the last long paper I wrote (with Don Dulaney) at Michigan, titled "A Stimulus-Response Analysis of Language and Meaning." When this usually enthusiastic man returned it without comment, or none that I can remember, I gathered that it lacked interest. I myself had thought that there was something very wrong with the paper because, although it was ingenious in its use of operant and respondent conditioning, it did not suggest a single experiment that I was interested in doing. The paper was essentially a translation of familiar aspects of language and meaning into the awkward terms of stimulus and response; it explained nothing and predicted nothing.

The theoretical terms of the Cognition Project, category, attribute, and criteriality, seized my imagination and filled my head with experiments on language and cognition that I really wanted to do. Jerome Bruner himself was an inspiration. He was a man who could convince a seminar that psychological problems of great antiquity were likely to be solved on that day by the group there assembled. After a few years I asked him to read a new paper; this one was called "Language and Categories." I have not kept his exciting note but I remember one phrase: "the deepest analysis of language I have ever read." He invited me to add it to *A Study of Thinking,* which was to be the Project's major book. He generously said I could make my paper a regular chapter in the book, which would have Bruner, Goodnow, and Austin as authors, or else place it separately as "Language and Categories: An Appendix by Roger Brown." I chose the second form.

It may be my imagination, fueled by forty years of the appointment process at Harvard, but I think my initial appointment may have been a kind of implicit "deal" between Allport and Bruner. Cognition certainly needed someone working on language, and social psychology needed someone to take Gardner Lindzey's place teaching the introductory course. Whether there was such a deal or not, my first assignments made social psychology and psycholinguistics my lifelong interests. For some reason, I have not done experiments in social psychology since my dissertation, but I love the content and have written two textbooks setting forth my organization of it. My research imagination seems only to work on problems involving language, but it has been productive there, resulting eventually in the longitudinal study of language acquisition in three preschool children we called Adam, Eve, and Sarah and in various papers on language processes.

* * *

Meantime, as they say, back at the raunch. Very little was going on. I located the tearooms at Harvard but did not take tea there because students from two large classes might have been upset to see me. I occasionally drove in to Boston's sedate Napoleon Club, the only gay bar I knew of, and stood at the back wall next to the fire escape ready to make a quick getaway in the event of a raid. There never was a raid, and no one attractive "never paid me no mind" at the back wall. My sentimental life was focused on Albert.

That was the year the magnificent Warren Milanov, Barbieri, and Björling *Trovatore* came out: I played it till the grooves gave out. I also ate many quarts of Brigham's coffee ice cream—the bachelor's solace in Cambridge.

I did make three new superior friends: Glen, Kevin, and Arthur. None of them in psychology; all in English and with exquisite taste in everything. The first time they saw my living room, which I had furnished with very great care, Arthur said: "What a horrible room!"

"What are those happy Italians singing about?" Glen asked as the three walked into my rooms on the day I got the recording. According to the libretto, no one in *Trovatore* has a single happy moment. But the singers do sound happy, as if it were enough to have the four greatest voices in the world and all the spaghetti you can eat.

Glen was the youngest of the three and the nearest to being sexually attractive. He knew the music was not intended to sound happy, but knew it only as a generalization about opera and not because he recognized *Trovatore*. Glen did not respond to music and openly said so. When he went to concerts or operas, he did it to accommodate his two friends who really liked the stuff.

I think Glen's missing gene for music must also be the gene for personal warmth. He was witty, hardworking, hospitable, and reliable, but he also was a bit cool. However, Glen was packaged with Kevin—very closely coupled they were for many years—and Kevin was a warm person. The problem was that Kevin was so devoted to Glen that what he gave to others was rather generic and so impersonal. But these two created the only lifelong, productive, happy, and, I think, monogamous male marriage in my experience. The cruel paradox of fidelity in male homosexuality is that the couples that stay together for longer than several months are mostly those that are sexually "open," but the few long-term couples that call themselves "happy" are the ones that achieve fidelity, the ones that are sexually closed.

"Shush! Milanov is about to produce one of her high pianissimo tones." Kevin's own tone was typically uxorious. He and Glen were the kind of spouses that chide one another in public, and rather rudely, and yet anyone can see how tight they are.

"Produce is certainly the word. It's not like singing at all. It's unearthly, like a beautiful sound given off by a Raphael painting." Arthur was the most artistic of the three, the most accomplished socially, and Arthur was unattached. He and I had a "go" at it once, just to square the circle, but it didn't work. Arthur used to be attached to Glen, but Glen and Kevin made a better match in that Glen was bossy and Kevin was submissive. However, they always lived as a threesome; one couple and a free radical looking for something to bond with.

"We look forward to meeting your friend Albert." Glen always said "Albert"; most people said "Al." Glen's "Albert" was pronounced with an odd intonation, higher on the first syllable. The effect to my ears was mildly mocking, as if to make fun of Albert's presumption in being known to me and his family by his full two-syllable name when most American men were content with abbreviations. Indeed, I think Glen took a mocking attitude toward Albert. I'm not sure why. Glen and Arthur and Albert too were all Jewish, but Albert was not a Harvard student and not at all assimilated to Cantabrigian ways.

"When is he coming?"

"On Sunday." It was the first week in June.

"Why don't you both have dinner with us?"

"Thanks, we will. He's heard about all of you and looks forward to meeting you. Albert likes to have a circle of friends. He's very sociable."

"You've had a good year here, wouldn't you say?" asked Glen. "You've been promoted to assistant professor, appointed head tutor in your department, had two papers accepted by journals, and started two long theoretical papers. I call that a good year."

Glen and Kevin and Arthur were all winding up their dissertations and had good job offers at, respectively, Boston College, Wheelock, and Boston University. But all three had bad cases of Harvard-itis. In speech, clothing, and values they were Harvard men and thought there were no *real* professors but Harvard professors. However, they had no Harvard prospects and couldn't see why I should have any either. I tried to remember this and to downplay my good fortune, but I didn't always feel like it; sometimes I felt like rubbing it in. In the end that broke up the friendship.

"Can you honestly say that you have been less happy here than you were at Michigan? Not to belittle Albert, but has his absence made such a great difference?"

I gasped at their lack of understanding. We had spent an entire year together and they had no sense that this was all essentially "time out" for me. The year lacked depth. The things that went well, the research, the writing, and the teaching, were all compensations, as were these three friends, but they were not advances on the main business of my life. What was that main business? It seemed to be to win Albert's wholehearted love. The year away had done none of the things I thought it might do. It had not broken the attachment or weakened it. It had simply been an interruption. My main concern had been that it should be *only* an interruption, that there would be a resumption. Probably it would be as difficult as ever, but it was the only thing, finally, that I felt was worth doing.

"Yes," I said. "Albert has made that great a difference."

* * *

When Albert arrived, he moved into a small street-level apartment on Bow Street in Cambridge quite near the Cognition Project, which was located in an old two-story frame house at the Massachusetts Avenue end of Bow Street. Nearby was a Catholic church which was headquarters for a rather sinister sect led by one Father Feeney. The members were all men and they dressed always in black suits, which gave them a Mafia look to us. We never knew what the sect was all about and were not curious enough to ask, but from time to time one heard a rumor that Father Feeney had been excommunicated.

Albert had no interest in interior decoration and he took the apartment because it came "furnished"—a bed, a couple of lamps and chairs, and a kitchen table. Albert added nothing to this bare minimum but stacks of books and papers.

Kirkland House, where I lived, was only a short distance away. It is one of the "river houses," which is the name given to Eliot, Lowell, Winthrop, and Dunster, as well as Kirkland. They are all in the same style of Georgian architecture, ivy-covered, and constructed of red brick. Several have handsome towers of azure blue or sapphire tipped with gold. Kirkland did not actually face on the river as most did, and my side looked out on a busy street and streetcar barns. It also sported no tower and was visually the least prepossessing of the river houses.

Still Kirkland was very impressive to me and to Al. It had a large junior common room with leather furniture and a grand piano and walls of fumed oak. It had a smaller senior common room, where the staff tutors socialized and had meetings and drank sherry, which came out of a sherry closet the key to which was held by the housemaster, Mason Hammond, a professor of classics. At Michigan we had not even heard the phrase "common room" and certainly had never been invited to have a sherry. At Michigan undergraduates lived in dormitories in rooms for two or three, with bunk beds and one washstand. Bathrooms and showers were shared by all the men in a corridor. I could not get over the fact that as a resident tutor I was given a private suite, consisting of a living room, bedroom, and bathroom (with a tub), and undergraduates lived nearly as well. Al's apartment, by comparison, looked crummy but he never seemed to mind.

After two years we moved in together to an apartment on Concord Avenue across from Observatory Hill and only a few blocks from Harvard Square, where the "T," or subway, had a stop. The apartment was not furnished and so we had to buy everything: dishes, pots and pans, beds, chairs, etc. Even to *think* of everything was a woeful strain on us. On Concord Avenue it became clear that Albert and I would always live more like graduate students than professors, because the work of buying property and making interior-decorating decisions held no appeal for us. We both needed faculty wives.

I thought Albert was worse than I was because he always wanted to own as little as possible. He lived like a merchant seaman who would always be prepared to ship out on short notice. I was always afraid he would. On the other hand, when we did buy something, his judgment was much better than mine. I could never see the item in context and so, left to myself, would buy something attractive enough on its own, but when brought home it would never "fit in." Not just aesthetically but physically. I have quantities of sheets and duvets and bedspreads which are either of king size, or queen size whereas the largest bed is just an ordinary double and, in making the bed, one has to try to fold under great stretches of fabric on the side next to the wall.

* * *

When someone is appointed to an assistant professorship at Harvard, he or she is promptly told there is no prospect of promotion, no tenure track for Harvard, and that is the near exceptionless truth. Yale is different in that there is some small possibility of promotion. When I was an assistant professor I visited Yale one day and went from office to office, paying short calls on junior faculty members, and was surprised at how much they bad-mouthed and belittled one another. At Harvard there was very little hostility among assistant professors; we spoke well of one another. The reason for the difference is, I think, that a zero-opportunity system is more comfortable than a low-opportunity system because the latter fosters intense competition.

In the last year of a Harvard term appointment (which for me was 1956-57), one's thinking changes. It turns out that you have been hoping that your case would be the exception; my case certainly felt exceptional to me and, while I never spoke of it and almost never thought it, in the end it turned out that I really could not imagine my department getting along without me, without my superb teaching and my administrative skills as head tutor and without my groundbreaking research. I had accepted every challenge, and tried to do everything well, in part to find out what I did best, because at that age you still don't quite know. I had found out, however, that experiments on psycholinguistics and writing on psycholinguistics were my own principal passions, and with the publication of "Language and Categories" in the Bruner book and of *Words and Things,* which I wrote in a sabbatical semester as assistant professor, much of American psychology would become interested in my subject. It did, but that did not keep Harvard from letting me go.

Albert was possibly going to get tenure at Boston University because, while his publications were few, his teaching was already famous. Still the decision on tenure for him was a long way off. It was certain that I was going to have to change universities, and my research reputation meant that I would be able to, but it was also likely that Albert would not have to and also would not be able to because teaching reputations have a strictly local value. Once again, then, we had a chance to think about whether we wanted to stay together.

"I don't think I will get tenure. Teaching alone is not enough; you have to have published."

"But not very much, with your teaching reputation."

"More than *Shakespeare Quarterly* abstracts. It would be embarrassing to offer nothing more."

"You'll have more; you'll have the Classic edition of *Twelfth Night,* edited by Albert Gilman and with an Introduction by Albert Gilman." Glen, now at Boston College, had a considerable reputation as a Shakespeare scholar and had been named general editor of a projected complete edition of Shakespeare's plays in paperback, one play to a book with some recognized authority as editor of each book. Along with one of the plays each book would include selected articles and commentaries from a variety of sources, as well as an Introduction by the editor.

"I can edit the play and pick the articles well enough, but I'm not sure I'm up to the Introduction. I was counting on you to help with the writing."

"I will if you supply the content."

"Even if the Introduction comes off it won't be enough; there has to be some original scholarship."

"Why don't we do something together? Something both psycholinguistic and literary. I have been thinking about formal and intimate pronouns of address like *tu* and *vous* in French, and I have asked students about cognate forms in Italian and Spanish and Russian and Greek and Latin, and every language seems to have them: what you might call 'T' and 'V' pronouns. Furthermore, though I don't have much to go on yet, the underlying semantic dimensions seem always to be the same: solidarity and power. A good case can be made that these are the basic dimensions of social relationship; solidarity or closeness would be the horizontal and power or status would be the vertical. If 'T' and 'V' forms are as universal as they appear to be, we have the interesting question: 'Why are they missing from English?' "

"They're not, or at least they weren't always. I think 'thou' and 'ye' are the equivalents. Shakespeare always uses both and I've seen references to whole monographs on Shakespeare's use of 'thou' and 'ye.' "

"Even more interesting! Why did English lose the contrast when other languages have not? There's bound to be a great paper in this. You could work on Shakespeare's uses and what happened in English history and I'd interview speakers of other languages."

"But you have to leave Harvard. You'll get plenty of offers, but I don't see how we can collaborate at a distance. Boston University or Tufts would probably be glad to get you, but I wouldn't let you go to a school like that. It would be a big step down and you would have a huge teaching load. Eventually Harvard is going to ask you back if you continue to make a splash."

"Swarthmore is my only hard offer so far, and it really appeals to me. Even though it's a small liberal arts college, some great psychologists have taught there; Solomon Asch, for instance. And the students are like Harvard students. It would be a different kind of life than Harvard but an appealing one. Except it's near Philadelphia and so a long way from you. So it's not the answer."

This was a conversation about staying together or separating, but it does not seem to belong to the same class as the conversations on that subject when we left Michigan. Had our heads at last come to govern our hearts? Not exactly. But we no longer had time for arguments over sex. I was in full career and giving all my time to research, writing, and teaching and wanting nothing else. My ambitions were limitless. I had no time for idle pastimes like sex. Well, actually I had sex, usually on Sunday morning and always with Albert, and it was neither lingering nor loving. I loved Albert but I expressed it in working with him and going to the theater and seeing our friends and summer travel.

Albert was less engrossed in his work but still very busy. He had not given up cruising; he never did. But it was limited in time and in venturesomeness. Just a few safe places for a few hours on some days. It did not bother me; in fact, I scarcely thought about it. After he got sick I felt grateful that he had not succumbed to my pressure but had his fun. Many times in the last month I longed to hear him say: "Well, I guess I'll go out for a while." But he no longer felt like it.

It was in these years (and they lasted a long time, from Al's arrival in Cambridge in 1953 until about 1964), when we gave least thought to love of any kind, that we loved one another best and were happiest. When I think about the times when we were closest they were not sex times at all. They were times of shared exaltation: hearing music, or seeing plays, or traveling, or just laughing over something funny.

We did not travel to the American Southwest until we had seen much of Europe, because we thought we had seen the American West in cowboy movies and that there was not much there for us. But movies and postcards do not capture the *immensity*. On first sight of the Grand Canyon we added it to the small list of sights that live up to one's greatest expectations: the Sahara, the Parthenon, Venice, the Bay of Naples—not much else that we had seen. Operas and plays are not disappointing in themselves but are in their performance, except once in a very long while.

We knew what to expect of *The Merchant of Venice*, but Olivier as Shylock at the Old Vic in London was a stunning surprise. We knew what to expect of *King Lear*, but not what Ralph Richardson would do with the line "O let me not be mad" on a Royal Shakespeare television tape. Beethoven's *Fidelio* was a familiar thrill, but Gwyneth Jones in her first Leonora at the Vienna *Staatsoper* stayed with us all our lives; I can even remember where we were sitting—a box on the right, over the stage.

It was Bayreuth in the 1950s, when Wieland Wagner was directing, that Albert pronounced "the greatest theater of any kind in the world," and we went many times to experience incomparable thrills. *Tristan und Isolde* in a banner performance with Nilsson and Windgassen, Böhm conducting, was so exciting it set nerves jumping all over your body. Most unforgettable, perhaps, was Maria Callas in *La Sonnambula* at the Edinburgh Festival. For the brilliant aria that ends the opera, "Ah, non credea mirarti," all the lights in the house were raised—an unprecedented thing to do—and Callas, beautiful in a brilliant white gown, stepped to the footlights and tossed off that impossible aria in death-defying cascades of tone. Andrew Harvey, in his wonderful novel *Burning Houses,* writes of the event and creates an after-performance backstage Callas who says: "Take that, Rosa Ponselle!" and from her bag draws a huge salami sandwich.

These are all "flashbulb memories" for me, memories that are exceptionally vivid, long-lasting, and detailed. A state of high emotion is the necessary condition. I have many more flashbulb memories for music than for drama. It may have been the other way around for Al. The important thing is that we could have such experiences in synchrony. It adds a great deal to have such an experience with someone you love. It is not a prerequisite that there be such a person there. It is possible to have solitary moments on this level. The other person is not necessary to produce the emotion, but the emotion, if it is shared with the other, creates a powerful meltdown or bond. Even one such experience can create a bond that will last for some years; many such experiences for the same two persons can almost fuse them into one.

Albert's brain cancer was diagnosed in 1989. Brain cancer followed lung cancer. It usually does. Metastasis to the brain from the lung is usual. He still had six months to live, what I wanted most was not just time but more moments of emotional fusion. We had several. One happy one that I remember well was Elizabeth Söderstrom singing the Marschallin in *Rosenkavalier*. We were sitting in the orchestra in the middle. Albert was on my right and some friend sat between us. The electricity jumped the gap.

For 1965 Al and I were both granted spring semester sabbatical leave. We had earned the sabbatical in the sense of having put in the requisite number of years of continuous duty, but a sabbatical is never quite automatic; you have to put in a request that includes the use you plan to make of the freed time. "Rest and recreation" is not an acceptable answer.

"What am I going to do for a whole semester? I don't have any scholarly project."

"They don't pay any attention to the project. You have to write something down, that's all. The sabbatical is owed you because of your years of continuous teaching."

"I wouldn't even know where to start."

"Why don't we write down something we can do together and might actually do: 'Further Studies in European Pronouns of Address.' We could add new languages to those already studied. Or we could check actual usage against what our informants told us. The project is very credible, since we already have published articles on the subject, both separately and jointly. We can say we will be working collaboratively."

"That's a good idea, but I thought we were planning to spend most of the time in England."

"We will. We have Eric and Michael there, and Mabel. Eric and Michael and Mabel were very funny, very camp English friends in the fashion trade whom we had met in earlier travels. I don't think we want to go to someplace where we have no friends."

"And can't speak the language."

"No, it definitely has to be England. In fact, mostly London. It will be wonderful to have the Royal Shakespeare and Royal Court companies and opera at Covent Garden and Sadler's Wells. All easily reached by subway."

"That's great, but how do we explain living in London when we plan comparative studies of pronouns of address?"

"Short trips to the Continent. Much easier from London than from the United States. The trips can be for data collection arranged for in advance with colleagues in other countries. Data collection need not take much time. The work of analysis can be in London. It's all reasonable, but in fact I do not think whoever reads these requests bothers about that level of detail."

"Since we will be living in London, shouldn't I add something relevant to Shakespeare? I can visit the Globe Theatre and go to Stratford when they put on plays I haven't seen."

"We certainly will want to do that, and you could mention the possibilities to people in your department, but my guess is that the written project will be stronger if we limit it to the single collaborative effort. It will look more serious, more like something we have thought about and will do." We *did* write the paper and "The Pronouns of Power and Solidarity" has become a foundation of the field called "Sociolinguistics."

In London we rented a furnished apartment on Dovehouse Street, which is in Kensington, just off the Fulham Road. It was not far from Eric and Michael, who had a penthouse with a small roof garden on Primrose Hill, and it was very close to Mabel, who had a cozy flat in Kensington. I remember the first dinner Mabel made for us, when I said, not quite seriously, "What is this creature we're eating? It's the best thing I've ever tasted."

"It's an ordinary scratching hen, luv." And it occurred to me that this was my first taste of a chicken that had never been frozen. Mabel was about forty, with bleached blond hair that was not quite sufficient to conceal her pink scalp. She squinted one eye even when she was not smoking, which was seldom. Al and I often took her to Covent Garden because she claimed to love opera, and the minute the curtain rose she fell dead asleep, but one minute before it fell some preconscious signal would awaken her and she would explode into applause, like a startled hen, and say, "Oh, darling, wasn't it marvelous!"

Eric was director of a clothing design firm for which both Mabel and Michael worked. Except for his knowledge of the arts, which was enormous, and his talent for design and his wit, he was a stereotypical English pouf, and he never pretended otherwise. I have noticed that Eric's in-your-face flaunting style is associated with personal courage in other areas, areas where it is admired. It was so in Eric's case. He was decorated for bravery in the Royal Air Force. He also had a long-term affair with another officer who was married. When they were together in close quarters Eric said he did not like looking at the wife's picture. I asked why he didn't turn her face to the wall and Eric said: "Darling, my face was turned to the wall."

Michael was Eric's lover and they lived together. Michael was only about thirty-five and a very campy young man. But then they were all in the "rag trade," as they called fashion design, and in that trade effeminate manners are hardly noticed. Mabel had been Eric's closest friend before Michael came on the scene and there was a little running tension there among the three.

Al and I lived in the midst of this London life and took an interest in the interpersonal emotions without seriously participating in them. We learned English manners. When turning down an invitation, you don't just say: "I'd like to come but, unfortunately, I'm busy on Tuesday." A few more layers of politeness, please. "Oh wonderful, I'd love to come. Let me just check my book. Damn! I have the worst luck. Tuesday is the day I promised Lord Bracknell to do Grand Rounds at the Maudsley. Can you possibly give me a raincheck?" Hospitality, we were explicitly told by both Eric and Mabel, must be promptly returned and in commensurate scale. London manners follow the same rules as American manners but are somewhat elevated in scale. To an American they seem more polite.

It was while we were living this life that I received copies of reviews of my first *Social Psychology*. They were all very favorable but one was unforgettable. M. Brewster Smith, a senior and respected social psychologist, had been asked to write an omnibus review of three new texts; one of the three was by Theodore Newcomb, who had been a professor at Michigan when I was a graduate student there. No one in social psychology was more admired than Professor Newcomb, so I figured his text for the sure winner in Brewster Smith's evaluation. Not so. The review came down very strongly for me. A little later Professor Newcomb wrote to say that, for his course in introductory social psychology, he had adopted, not his own brand-new book, but mine. He ended the letter most endearingly: "I am trying to think of some way that I can claim you."

That was the beginning of the triumphal progress of *Social Psychology*, a progress that continued for some years. It is just as well that I was in London with my friends in the rag trade, because their outsiders' view somewhat kept my egotistical joy in perspective.

One of the reasons Albert and I had chosen to spend our sabbatical in England was that York University had invited me to accept an honorary degree. It is unusual for someone as young as I was then (forty) to be offered an honorary degree. It is more unusual for such an invitation to come from a country other than one's own. To receive the degree you must attend the commencement ceremonies, and this I was strongly inclined to do.

We planned a tour by car of England and Scotland which would include a two-week stay at York at commencement time. I had invitations to lecture at Oxford, Cambridge, Edinburgh, Leeds, and the London School of Economics. Albert did not have any such invitations but was enthusiastic about using the universities to guide a tour of Britain. I felt relaxed about the plan because I had two polished lectures, just two, but that was as many as I would need anywhere.

In those days I had not yet been "psyched out" and was a good lecturer. I knew how to build tension in an audience, how to use wit so it would seem spontaneous, and when to let the argument climax. The Harvard *Confidential Guide* to courses called me "one of the freshest lecturers in the college."

In the beginning I used notes on three-by-five cards but eventually realized that I did not need them any more than Toscanini needed a baton. Professor Bruner used to marvel at this accomplishment and say: "I don't know how you unfold a complex argument entirely without notes."

In preparation it was necessary to decide on the order of major events and to know what things were subordinate and what things superordinate, but it was a mistake to work out actual sentences. In a good lecture the speaker thinks about content as he speaks, not wording. Thinking as you speak makes the intonations, timing, and word choice better than they ever are if a lecture is written out and memorized. In addition, the audience enjoys the tension of a high-wire act without a safety net.

At Edinburgh I had my best reception. The audience was huge—which always helps. The introduction was deeply knowledgeable about my work and delivered by a graduate student with enormous honest enthusiasm.

Al never came to my lectures because it would have made me nervous and would have bored him. I generally dodged out of post-lecture receptions and dinners and hurried back to spend the evening with him. During the lecture he wandered about the town and did sight-seeing. In Edinburgh there is much to see. The castle high above the town, the colorful changing of the guard, and everywhere the monuments that look like thistle turned to stone. I got back to our hotel much inflated by my success and eager to tell Al about it.

"I wish you had come. It went really well. The best so far, I think." Al's face was buried in his pillow but now he turned it up to me. It was sadly battered and swollen.

"Good God, what happened to you?"

"Someone beat me up and chased me back to the door of the hotel."

"Who was it? Have you called the police?"

"Can't call the police. I'm just glad he doesn't know my name or the room number. I tried to pick him up. In fact I did pick him up. We went back to his room. I should have known something was wrong. He was too good to be true. A big solid Scotsman with red hair and in kilts. He turned out to be straight and a faggot-hater. My antennae must have been thrown off by his Scots accent. Anyway, when I had done my thing—which he gave every sign of enjoying—he hit me in the face and bellowed: 'This is what I think of fucking cocksuckers.' Luckily I was fully dressed and got out the door and headed back to the hotel before him."

I'm afraid I did not feel pity but disgust, and anger at having my brilliant day ruined. "I thought you knew better than to cruise in a foreign country. I had a beautiful day and you've ruined it."

"You bastard! Can't you see I've been beat up and humiliated? And all you think of is yourself."

"Why do you have to take such chances? Why couldn't you come to the lecture or just visit the castle?"

"I'm not your faculty wife, content to bask in your glory. I don't even share in it because no one must know that we are connected."

We screamed at one another most of the night. And on the long train ride from Edinburgh back to York, neither said a word. Edinburgh must have been the worst bust-up since I remember it so clearly, but there were many others in that year, when we had more time than usual to hurt one another.

* * *

I am not quite sure how alcohol came into our lives. For me it was at first a means of dealing with performance anxiety on the road. I got so I could not easily fall asleep on the night before a "big lecture" and it would seem to me that my talk was below standard when I did not get eight good hours.

I have heard that Franco Corelli retired from the operatic stage because he was "psyched out" by this kind of performance anxiety. Whether or not this was true of Corelli, I can understand how it might happen to any performer who has come to count on enthusiastic audience applause; and the fact that this was true of me indicates that there was as much showman as scientist in my makeup.

Eventually I developed performance anxiety over the "little" lectures on home ground that are simply class meetings and settled into the pattern that lasted for years–a controlled alcoholism. I drank only at night, as a somnolent to wipe out anxiety, never in the daytime, never for pleasure except as an elimination of worry. A doctor once asked me if I considered myself an alcoholic:

"Perhaps, if the definition is medical, since I may drink too much for the health of my body. But there is also a social-psychological aspect. Does the controlled drinking I do harm anyone? It does not harm my students, I'm sure, since it has worn off before morning. Nor do I think it harms any aspect of my work. It may even be a necessary aid." After Albert died I drank the same amount as before but felt that I had ceased to be an alcoholic since my drinking disturbed no one. In his lifetime, however, it disturbed him very much, and since I continued in the face of that disturbance I was then definitely an alcoholic.

In O'Neill's *Long Day's Journey into Night,* one of the men says that Mary Tyrone seems to take morphine in order to escape her husband and two sons. She becomes a living ghost in the New London fog, unreachable by any of them. That's how it feels to be alone with a person drinking–even a little–and why it is an unbearable situation. The drinker withdraws–willfully–from oneself and into a fog. The one not drinking becomes very expert at detecting such withdrawal; slightly slurred speech or a comment not really relevant are enough to give away the fact that the whole person is no longer with you.

I think I began drinking in the evening before Al did and I think he then took it up to exorcise the ghost beside him. We both escaped the worries of the day and also one another. Al used to call the hours from four to six in the afternoon the "difficult hours." No business engaged us and it was too early for dinner or entertainment. We had only one another and that was not enough. It is hard to say why it was not enough, but I think it had to do with the sexual and romantic dissatisfaction each of us felt.

We did our weekly grocery shopping at the Stop and Shop supermarket—a hateful chore. Putting away the groceries one night, Albert said, pointing at two quart bottles of Gordon's vodka, "Look at that. You know what we've become? Two old drunks."

"It's not that bad. We get a little high, not drunk, and we both function well at work and socially."

"We're going through half a gallon every week. We're going to bed half-stoned most nights. It's a miracle one of us hasn't fallen and broken something or set fire to the house."

"Well, let's try to cut back some. We can do it gradually."

"That won't work. I've made some inquiries and signed up to go into the detoxification unit at Faulkner Hospital in two weeks."

"Without telling me? I don't think I could go into a detox unit. You live there, you know, and all alcohol is stopped. I'd be afraid I might have seizures—like Tennessee Williams did when he had to have an emergency operation."

"They have medication to prevent seizures. The people at Faulkner say that a complete stop with a week of detoxification is the only thing that works. And after that you have to go to Alcoholics Anonymous meetings. A lot of them at first."

"I don't think I could do it, Albert. You know how I hate hospitals and the idea of stopping cold turkey scares me. And I could never find the time to go to a lot of stupid meetings."

"You can do what you like. I'm going into Faulkner in two weeks." And Albert walked out of my room and into his own.

I felt deserted; "sola, perduta, abandonnata," as Manon Lescaut says. After all our years doing everything together, he could contemplate an independent change of course that might separate us forever. It had always been I who had threatened and attempted separation, I who had stormed out at night. Al had never threatened anything. And that was what made his plan terrifying. Whatever he planned he always had the strength to carry out. Besides, he was not threatening to leave me, only to break a self-destructive pattern.

I was free to detoxify with him if I could. But I knew I could not and I was filled with panic that I might lose him.

I made a private plan. While Albert was at Faulkner I would carry out a detoxification program of my own, a program I thought I could execute. Since living with Albert was, I judged, a major cause of stress for me, I should in his absence have the strength to reduce my bedtime medication. I would gradually cut back the alcohol to almost but not quite zero. I did not, in my thinking, commit myself to a goal of zero medication in one week. That idea scared me. But small reductions every night would bring me close to zero, perhaps, I imagined, somehow to zero itself. And so, when Albert returned free of his addiction, I would be almost, if not quite, free of mine and he would see that I too was reformed.

I drove him to Faulkner. The place and the program did not look so bad, and I almost changed my mind and stayed with him. At the end of the week he was free of alcohol and I was almost, but not quite, free. As part of a general physical exam in the hospital Al had a chest Xray, which revealed some abnormality in one lung—something to follow up but not worry about.

I really don't think Al was ever tempted to drink again. He was very responsive to behavior therapies, it seemed, and just as some twenty years earlier the Smoke Enders program had enabled him to give up cigarettes, so now a week of detox and the AA program enabled him to give up drinking. He greatly enjoyed AA meetings and went to even more of them than the program recommended. He went at noontime and during the difficult hours from four to six and evenings and weekends. In order to be with him, I started accompanying him; and while I never could figure out why AA worked (and it certainly didn't work for me), the meetings were enjoyable.

We had certain favorites. There was a meeting at noontime on Beacon Hill which mostly drew well-dressed professional men, doctors and lawyers and executives. It was quite dramatic to hear these pin-striped gentlemen spill their guts in confession of alcoholic horrors. Several were former students of mine and in a very friendly way offered to serve as my sponsors. There was the West Church group, which was mostly made up of young men plus Albert and me. Most of the young men were named Kevin and their tales of addiction were sadly similar. Neither Albert nor I ever made a "confession" and groups exerted no pressure to do so. One time, however, the leader decided we should go all around the room and state our names and problems. I was not keen on doing this and when it came my turn I'm afraid I said: "I'm addicted to drugs and alcohol and my name is Kevin."

AA meetings were just a novel form of social life and theater to both Al and me. He did give up drinking, totally and for the rest of his life; he had stopped with the hospital detox program and never started again. I don't think the AA meetings had anything to do with it. I attended the same meetings and my nightly intake of alcohol crept back up to its former level and stayed there.

We even tried to use AA meetings to entertain our friends. Cheryl, who taught at Johns Hopkins University, spent an unforgettably unseasonal Christmas Eve with us. Her idea had been to spend the magic hours listening to Bach chorales at Emmanuel Church. We nixed that in favor of the AA Grand Holiday Marathon, in which all the alcoholics in Boston got together to support one another in not drinking through the Season of Temptation. The most bloodcurdling and histrionic confessions were trotted out; not at all the right thing for Christmas Eve, Cheryl felt.

Every summer Dodie Pucci, the well-known painter, spent a week with Albert and me at Provincetown. Though Dodie now lived in Germany and was very much a European woman, she had been born and grown up in Everett, Massachusetts, where her mother still lived. She had been Al's student at Boston University. At Al's funeral in 1989 Dodie said: "He was the first brilliant person I had ever met; it makes such a difference." The freshness of that sentence was characteristic; Dodie never took a nine to five job or joined the middle-class, but lived always as an artist; and that may be why she has stayed free of cliché.

We dragged Dodie one summer to a session of the Provincetown AA, thinking it ought to be especially interesting. She tried to be as inconspicuous as possible and avoided meeting anyone's eyes—not at all her usual style. Afterwards she explained to our blunter sensibilities: "I felt like such a hypocrite, pretending to be something I'm not. Something very serious for them."

It was more boredom than moral scruple that caused us to stop going to AA. But in less than a year we did. Albert was dry forever and I had my controlled limited addiction–also forever.

* * *

Before I describe the last events of our lives together, which are very terrible for me, let me remember that much of the time Albert and I were a Laurel and Hardy comedy. Al was Ollie and I sometimes called him that, and I was Stan and he sometimes called me that. Laurel and Hardy, when I was a boy, could make me laugh until my stomach hurt. When Al and I developed into the same sort of inept innocents, our escapades sometimes made us laugh almost that hard. We grew into the habit of saying in concert: "Here's another fine mess you've gotten me into."

Albert was Ollie not by virtue of girth but because he had the same sort of "take charge" manner, the same superior knowledge of how things worked, the same way of issuing peremptory orders to poor dim-witted, distractable Stan. Our intentions were always benign and our manners courtly, but we wreaked unimaginable damage on ourselves and others because in execution we, like Laurel and Hardy, were inept. The world, both human and physical, was too complex for us, just as it was for them.

I always thought of us as Stan and Ollie when Albert had to ask me to do something personal for him–like tying his black tie for formal dress. In the first place, he didn't like asking. Nor did he like the close face-to-face contact. And I always seemed to choke him or lose the knot or get one end longer than the other. Laurel and Hardy in the movie *Way Out West* have a scene where Ollie has around his neck a woman's precious locket–never mind how come–and Stan is to remove it by pulling it over Ollie's head. That is not easy. Ollie winces and groans and gives orders as the chain digs into his fat neck and multiple chins and catches on his nose, and Stan just applies more muscle. In the end, Ollie's detachable collar is off and his shirt torn but the locket still in place. In spite of all the indignities and injuries he has suffered, including a red nose and swollen eye, Ollie only expresses a kind of patient exasperation. Stan, as usual, is just puzzled.

Albert and I had many such scenes. Almost always when close cooperation was called for: fumbling with coupons at the supermarket checkout, assembling a bookcase, hooking up a TV, or trying to give a party. At one dinner party a rude guest asked: "Have they ever entertained before?"

My own favorite Stan and Ollie skit came on our cruise of the Galápagos Islands. The tour group included a young family from Wellesley, the Nelsons, Ron and Gail, prosperous and good-looking, and their two high-school-aged sons who were both headed for Harvard. The parents were so very Banana Republic that when Ron skipped on deck the first day in the islands I said: "What beach are we taking today, Ron?"

This family that lived so near Cambridge and had also a certain knowledge about collegiate life diluted the anonymity we usually felt on tours. In their heterosexual perfection, they made us feel our deviance as a male couple more sharply than we usually did.

The sons had their own cabin on the deck below us but Ron and Gail were just next door. The little ship was unique in having no locks on cabin doors and guests were reminded every day to put valuables in the ship's safe, but theft, we learned, was not the only peril for those at sea. I remember still the look of the cabins from the outside. They were identical except for their placement, wooden slats painted green with brass hardware. Ron and Gail had the corner cabin next to the ladder while Albert and I were one cabin down the line.

The second day in the islands I lay in my bunk reading when Albert staggered in, white and trembling: "Oh my God, I opened the wrong door and there they were, Ron and Gail, having sex!"

"Jesus, what did you say?"

"Nothing. I couldn't speak. Just groped my way back out the door. It was a nightmare."

"Never mind, Ollie. It could happen to anyone. It's *crazy* not having locks on the cabin doors." I didn't ask *how* they were having sex for fear it would exacerbate Al's panic.

The next afternoon, at almost the same time, Albert literally fell into our cabin. He clapped his hand to his flushed forehead. "I can't believe it! I did it again and they were at it again! I must be losing my mind."

That evening at dinner Ron paled when Albert came in and squared his jaw as if he might have to have "words." Albert apologized profusely and said he thought he might have a touch of seasickness. He would have liked to say "I didn't *see* anything," but of course he couldn't. After a bit Ron and Gail found it possible to laugh and tell him to forget it.

Next morning, right after breakfast, Albert fell over our threshold and stuttered: "I did it again, I actually did. Lock me up or something."

Stan couldn't help giggling this time. "They'll think we're selling tickets." That set both Stan and Ollie howling with laughter at the two rabbits next door.

That was the best encounter with the Nelsons but not the last. As we went through customs in New York, Ron said, and my memory for this is verbatim, "I don't know how you two boys go down on your campuses, but on a trip you are really a 'trip.'" He actually did call us "boys," and that is what people call Laurel and Hardy in their movies.

Both of the Nelson sons did go to Harvard, two years apart, and each came to my office in his turn, respectfully introduced himself, and reminded me that we had once taken a cruise together. I did notice that neither took a course with me.

* * *

Whatever may be said of our mental health, Al and I had good physical health for more than sixty years, until about 1988. In fact, we had generally good luck, no hurricane damage, no fires, no gay-bashing, no arrests, no social diseases. Of course we knew that some or all of these things were coming. They happened to everyone else and our turn must come. At that time I felt very guilty about Al because he seemed unhappy and that was partly because I continued my drinking pattern and partly because he was not getting the recognition he deserved at Boston University. I used to say a little prayer: "God, be good to Albert and don't worry about me." So much for the efficacy of prayer. Our serious troubles started with me but when his came they were far worse.

In a routine physical exam I was discovered to have prostate cancer and so scheduled for a prostatectomy. My reactions to my own health problems, even those that are life-threatening, suggest that the cast of my mind is truly psychological, even social-psychological. With the prostate cancer, the first serious problem, I was more interested in the effect of the news on Albert than I was in whether I would live or die. Why the interest? From his reaction I could perhaps judge accurately whether he had forgiven my transgressions against him. Was his forgiveness for me more important and more ambiguous than life or death? Apparently so.

Some years later, when Albert had died and Grant was the most important person on earth to me, I had a heart attack and a multiple coronary bypass, and my main interest in that event was whether it would bring Grant rushing to my bedside. It didn't. And there have been other events since, but what's the use of all these close calls if the interpersonal information they provide is always disappointing?

I have also noticed that interpersonal information is dominant for me over spectacular nonpersonal events and scenery. Al and I made some exotic trips in the last ten years of his life: the Warsaw Pact nations, all of them; the Galápagos Islands, Peru, and Machu Picchu; Israel and Egypt; Morocco; and, the last, Japan and Bangkok. We did all the traveling in group tours because the work of travel in out-of-the-way places had become too much for us.

If you have a tour group you have group dynamics. And I always found that I could not keep my mind on the scenery because I was too interested in what was going on in the group, even though these were temporary groups with no shared past and no future. As you flew back home you could feel the spell lifting, individuals passing out of mind; but when I was a member of a group, the Valley of the Kings could not hold my attention. It may be so for everyone, or only for psychologists, or only for very self-involved people.

The cancer had not metastasized beyond the prostate and the doctor cheeringly reported: "No further treatment is required at this time." I must have heard the last three words, since I can recall them, but the way I processed the sentence is: "No further treatment is required—a complete cure!" Only months later Al had surgery for lung cancer; the disease was discovered from a routine chest Xray taken when he was in the detox program at Faulkner Hospital. After his surgery, successful like mine, we heard the sentence we had heard before: "No further treatment is required at this time," and processed it once again as happy news of a complete cure. It must be something some subtle psycholinguist has put into medical school training. The final phrase "at this time" is not noted when the big news is up front. In less than six months Al's cancer required further treatment; mine did not for more than four years, but in the end it did. *At the time*, however, neither did.

I was in a panic about having to go into a hospital. Patients were forbidden to bring any of their own medications and told that the hospital would supply everything necessary. What about my terrible secret, the sleeping potion of vodka which I had now taken without fail every night for many years? I was certain I could not sleep without it, so certain that I had never tried. In a hospital alcohol was *strengst verboten*. I thought it likely that a sudden unknowing cutoff would send me into convulsions as a cutoff of his drugs had done with Tennessee Williams.

In desperation I went in for smuggling. A vodka bottle of any size, I thought, would be detected. Probably they searched patients on a daily basis. I noticed that some patients had been allowed to bring in Selsun, an over-the-counter antacid, that was put up in opaque blue plastic bottles. And so I emptied the contents of a Selsun bottle down the drain at home and filled it with Absolut. If you did not unscrew the cap and sniff it, it would be taken for Selsun. I surreptitiously swigged it and slept well even on the first night after the operation.

Selsun bottles are small and I needed a confederate on the outside to bring me a refill. It could not be Albert who, as a recovering alcoholic in AA, could not condone doing it. It could not be any of our friends because of the shame of revealing myself to be a certain kind of alcoholic. That left only Edwige, our housekeeper, who already knew what kind of alcoholic I was, and did not take it seriously since it was very limited. Still she would not do it. It was against the hospital's rules and if something went wrong with me because of the vodka she could never forgive herself. So I had to get uncharacteristically tough: "Edwige, do you want to keep your job or not?" With great guilt, she did it. And His Lordship slept.

"You'll be discharged tomorrow," the resident said. I'd only been in the hospital three days and was hooked up by the penis to an external catheter of some complexity which voided my urine.

"You must be kidding! I have no idea how to work the catheter. No one has shown me even once and it's bound to be dangerous."

"Oh, you'll learn how to do it." And he walked out. I was in a panic and called Al. "They're putting me out tomorrow and I'll have to be catheterized for at least a week, but I've no idea how to monitor levels, change the bag, or arrange the hose and neither of us is any good at mechanical things." Al's panic was twice as great as mine. He imagined me, half-stoned at night, tripping over the hose, and possibly killing myself. So he called his older sister Mollie in New York, who was chiefly concerned (as was Albert himself) about how my coming home would affect him. She advised him to call the head of the hospital and tell him there was no one at home to look after me.

"I'll sue the hospital if you send him tomorrow," Albert screamed over the phone. The residents, when they heard the story, seemed puzzled by the relationship between the two of us, which certainly sounded intense, though hardly loving. I took more Selsun than usual that night and fancied that one nurse kept sniffing my breath.

The hospital still planned to send me home the next day but gave me until noon. By the grace of God, the nurse who had charge of getting me ready was a kind and patient person. She spent a full two hours teaching me how to handle all aspects of the catheterization process. I knew I had to get it right and so did not mind at all that she and I had to throw my penis back and forth and put on rubber tubing and take it off and spill urine everywhere. After I got home I wrote her a note of thanks, the only time I have ever written such a note to a nurse, or felt like it.

I had recovered from my operation by the time Al's diagnosis of lung cancer was certain and a date set for surgery. I was more frightened than I had been of anything in my life. He was the primary person in my life and had been so for as long as I could remember. I could not imagine living without him. This was true even though we had not had sex, let alone made love, for some years.

My work got all my attention, except for the occasional male graduate student on whom I developed a crush. The greatest of these was my crush on James Kulik, with whom I wrote "Flashbulb Memories." Daryl Bem once said of Jim: "I am always impressed with Jim Kulik, but I never know whether it's because of his abilities or the way he looks." I think it's both. I use Jim's real name as an exception because he knows about my crush and, in later years, we talked about it and he always returned nothing less and nothing more than affection and admiration.

I never had sex with any of my students, never even came on to one, but I guess my infatuations were pretty obvious. Albert always knew, and in Jim Kulik's case so did his roommate. I had called with some exciting news about our data and I overheard the roommate relay the news to Jim in exaggeratedly fluttering female tones.

In the spell of a crush I did nothing but imagined much. Not sex. But another sort of life: romantic-age mates in a convertible on an open road. Speed, vistas, open air–and loving young buddies. Those have always been the constituents of this fantasy. Very different from Albert and myself doing our separate class preparations in our separate small bedrooms on Sunday afternoons.

Albert never had crushes as far as I ever noticed. He did have some outside impersonal sex, always. For a long time, as I have said, he and I had sex about once a week, usually on Sunday morning. It was neither loving nor exciting but mechanical and dutiful. It was Al who put a stop to it and he did it for me. It was the only sex I was having or seeking and he saw, as I did not, that I was using up the time of life in which I might hope to attract someone, anyone, and that my marriage kept any such away. The decision did not change things because I did not know of any easy way to meet attractive younger men. I did not know how to use escorts until after Albert's death. Instead I foolishly took his dictum as an expression of personal distaste for intimacy with me and added it to my list of grudges against him.

After Albert got his diagnosis of lung cancer, but before his operation, the relation between us was very strained. His way of dealing with the bad news was to try to be occupied socially every evening. His circle of friends liked to dine out but I did not. Had I had the foresight to realize what remorse I would suffer if he should die, I would have done whatever he liked and stayed always with him, but I did not and chose instead to stay at home and knock out my terror with vodka. I tried to be in bed, preferably asleep, by the time Al got home so as not to confront him with a ghost. Sometimes, however, he was unexpectedly early, and then there were terrible scenes. The worst of these stays in memory, excruciatingly painful. I was still in the living room when Al came home and he at once saw through my pretense of sobriety, hearing blurred speech and seeing a glazed stare. Then, watched closely, I tried to steer a straight line into my bedroom but stumbled over a chair and fell flat. Al screamed: "You filth! You scum! When I have cancer too!" My vodka put me out for about four hours. I got up and walked shakily into the kitchen and found what I knew would be there—a note in Al's childishly small but hysterically punctuated handwriting: "You rotten son of a bitch! You dirty bastard!" And so on. I sat down at the table with my head in my arms and cried and cried. And even so it was not the last time.

* * *

Albert's operation was a horror. It left his poor chest looking like something in a slaughterhouse. And it was done shortly after the worst quarrels of our life together.

Each night I came to his hospital bedside hoping for some sign of forgiveness and dreading that he would deliver instead a blast of hatred. He did neither. Sitting beside his bed, wrapped in a white nightgown that looked like a toga, he was grimly silent, stoical. Rebecca, a dear friend for many years, said he never looked handsomer nor more powerful and that was right. He might have been Coriolanus refusing to show his terrible wounds or tell what he had endured. His sister Mollie wanted to visit from New York, and he said he would like to have her there, which sounded as if he felt otherwise alone.

"Is the food terrible?" I asked.

"It's all right."

"What can I bring you?"

"Nothing."

"Do you have any pain?"

"No."

"I could have a cot moved in and sleep here if you want me to."

"I don't. You may as well go home. There's nothing to do here."

And I would go home. Not daring to touch him or even to approach closely. His austere manner and failure to look in my face seemed to forbid any familiarity. It was easier when Tilly was there. He almost smiled for her.

"Albert, I talked to our sister Pauline today. She's the same as ever; I don't know how she keeps on. She says she wakes up from her afternoon nap amazed to be still alive. And when she moves everything in her body hurts. Then she takes one pill, just one. What it is I can't imagine. And soon she's ready to go out dancing. And she goes to Dreamland with a couple of her girlfriends, and dances until midnight. She always has men who want to take her home, but she doesn't let them unless they are exceptionally attractive. I wish I had half her vitality. And looks. She still has those sparkling eyes and perfect skin. You and she, Albert, were always the ones with the looks in the family!"

"You look wonderful, Mollie. In the picture at Jack's wedding you looked like a queen."

"Albert, if I cut up this steak for you, would you eat a little bit? You've got to eat to get your strength back. I admit it doesn't look terribly appetizing. Why doesn't Roger go out now and get some brisket and that good bread at the deli? And maybe a piece of cheesecake?"

"No, I don't want anything."

When Albert came home he still did not talk much but we had our routine that forced cooperation: the weekly grocery shopping, the visits and dinners with friends. I never stayed away now but went everywhere with them. And I was very careful to cut my sleeping potion to an absolute minimum and never take it until he was asleep. Gradually he grew stronger. When he finally went out cruising my eyes were wet with gratitude. He never let me touch him anymore and of course he did not touch me.

* * *

We taught our courses in the spring term of 1989 and planned a summer trip on the grandest scale ever: six weeks in the Far East, including Japan, Hong Kong, China, Thailand, and Bali. The events in Tiananmen Square scratched China from the itinerary, and that was a great disappointment, but total time remained constant as new stops were substituted.

I never saw Albert so excited about a trip as he was about this one. He felt that he had to get his doctor's permission to make it, since it was only months after lung surgery. The doctor said, "Yes, go. By all means, go," and we set forth, both having passed through and survived cancer. Al had a little dizziness, but the doctor thought that was probably Ménière's syndrome, a common problem of the inner ear, and not serious.

We called Marian and Joan in San Francisco, who were thrilled about the trip.

"Why don't you stop and spend some time with us on your way out?"

"The starting date for the tour is May 23, which is just two days after Roger finishes at Harvard. So we thought we'd have our visit with you on the way back in July."

"That'll be great. We have Anna Jane visiting early in June and then we can look forward to seeing you in July as the main event of the summer."

The tour group did not look very promising at the introductory cocktail party and dinner. There was Maureen O'Day, a Southern girl traveling with her mother, who immediately looked to us to provide the "fun" on this journey. The tour guide was young and, we were sure, gay and seemed worried that we would break his cover. Plus a gaggle of women who couldn't wait to shop in Hong Kong and get a bargain on jade in Bangkok.

The flight on Singapore Airlines was fabulous. Stewardesses in long silk robes gave everyone a miniature bejewelled calculator as a souvenir. The bathrooms had shelves of colognes including Eau Sauvage, and the meals were served in many courses with linen napkins and beautiful wines.

In Tokyo, our first stop, we first felt some disappointment in our response to the Orient. It was hard to see why; the Buddhas were big and the trains were fast. Al put his finger on the problem: insufficient background. In Europe we always had a network of associations, musical and literary, that made any scenery romantic.

"Think of the English countryside, for instance. Not very different from Ohio, really. But we think of it as divided up into moors and heaths and fens and so on, haunted by the ghosts of the Brontë sisters, Wordsworth, Hardy, Britten and so on, so that there is hardly a meaningless tuft of grass in the country. But for us Japan is just all Japan with nothing to differentiate one part from another but the things on the surface today and, impressive as these are, they are less so than the deep net laid down in our lifetimes by Europe."

It was in Japan that one member of the tour took me aside and asked me if Al was feeling okay. She had noticed certain things.

"When we are in a crowd he just steamrolls ahead, looking neither to the right nor the left, and maintaining a steady, quite fast pace. Mostly people get out of his way but I have seen him occasionally knock into someone as if he hadn't seen them. And yesterday, getting on the subway, he stopped at the doorway and sort of hopped around as if he did not quite know when to step ahead. It's the same on escalators and trains. There's that odd hesitation and nervous look."

"I haven't noticed anything special on the trip, but that's probably because I'm used to Al's problems with balance and coordination. He had them before he came on the trip, as well as a feeling of dizziness, and he asked his doctor about them. The doctor wasn't sure but said it was probably Ménière's syndrome, which is a problem of the organs of balance in the inner ear. It is fairly common—my mother had it for a while—and it goes away spontaneously."

"I hope that's right. Have you noticed he looks sad or just 'out of things' quite often? Of course he's also very funny sometimes."

"I think that's just Al's disposition."

In Bangkok I got sick. I was lying on my bed after lunch, reading Virginia Woolf's *Mrs. Dalloway*. I had been reading and rereading *Mrs. Dalloway* throughout the tour to cleanse my ears of the tour guide spiels and the tourist wiseacres. On this day, however, something went wrong with my reading and a single phrase went around again and again without yielding up its meaning. I went unconscious and woke up in the Bangkok city hospital with a Thai neurologist asking my name and age and the name of the president of the United States. I had had a seizure—the first ever—and they called it "late onset epilepsy" but never did discover the cause. Not the fault of the hospital, which was very good.

The hospital insisted I stay two days and so the tour had to go on without me—us, as Al of course stayed with me. He came to my bedside and said, unforgettably: "In a way I'm glad this happened because I have to go back and find out what's wrong with me." I had not realized that he knew from the inside that something serious was wrong with him. Only two days before on the tour bus he made the group laugh by saying: "When are we going to visit the famous sex industry of Bangkok?"

The leader of the tour arranged an immediate flight back for us. We stayed just one night in San Francisco and heard from Marian and Joan all the variations that are possible on the sentence: "It's probably nothing serious."

* * *

The lung surgeon's "at this time" in the sentence "No additional treatment is required at this time" had run out and he now added the terrifying: "When lung cancer metastasizes, it is usually to the brain." And so it was now with Albert: to the cerebellum, which controls balance, and coordination, as does the inner ear, but centrally and gravely. From the cerebellum further tumors must be expected in the brain, and soon. The diagnosis was a death sentence.

"I do not care so much for myself. I just wish we had been able to get along better."

"I could not have loved you more if—" My sentence broke off because my voice quavered out of control but also because I did not know what to put after the "if." If what? There was what I might have done—put him first always, been selfless. And there was what he might have done—loved me as I wanted to be loved. I was probably choked by the realization that neither condition was controllable, that there had been no voluntary counterfactuals, that there never had been an alternative.

"What do you want to do in the time we have left? We can do anything you want."

"I'm going to teach my fall Shakespeare course; there isn't anything else I want to do. But there's not going to be any social withdrawal, Roger. We'll need all the help we can get."

In the three months that followed Al did teach his course. Incredibly, he graded the last paper days before the ambulance came to take him to the hospital. He had no pain and he slept every night without medication. He also did not go back to drinking. He did not cruise at all and I ached for the days when his doing so had tortured me. Just once I asked if I could do something for him sexually and he said: "Are you kidding?"

I had heard that when death approaches couples draw closer together than they have ever been. I hoped for that to happen to us but it did not. I subordinated every selfish concern and did whatever Albert wanted, when he wanted anything, but he moved no closer to me. Whether to punish me or just because it was his nature, he seemed determined to die with just that space between us that had always been there.

Just once he broke down a little and almost cried. We were driving home after a Sunday evening supper with our closest friends. He had been silent all evening and so had most of us; the thought in everyone's mind was that there could not now be many more such "family evenings." I clicked on the radio and it was Gwyneth Jones singing the *Liebestod*. I started sobbing and Al said, his voice shaking for once: "Turn it off. I feel it too."

One weekend loomed so very dreary that we felt we had to get out of town. The weather was gray and drizzly and all our friends were either out of town or otherwise engaged. We took the shuttle to New York and stayed one night at a hotel that our friend Barry recommended to us.

The hotel had been redecorated in a way that was both handsome and absurd. Every employee was dressed entirely in black. It was not permitted to move anything in the lobby because the placement, as well as color and design, of every table and chair contributed to a space conceived as sculpture.

The room consisted of two alcoves with a bed in each, as well as a gold pen and small pad with which to record whatever inspirations might visit one at night. The bathroom was all glass: dazzling to look at but no place at all for such things as toothbrushes and shaving cream.

Whatever moved—drawers, closets, cabinets—moved by some well-concealed mechanism. Albert spent the first half-hour plaintively calling Rosemary, in housekeeping; it became informal "Rosemary" through simple repetition. "Rosemary, how do you turn the bathroom light on?" "Rosemary, we can't get the clothes closet door open." For that one night, at least, the matched alcoves and the comedy of the room brought us together.

In the last few weeks Al sometimes felt that he wanted to enjoy once again simple foods he had loved when he was a boy. Rebecca, though she was a grand gourmet cook, loved indulging these desires. "Rebecca, what I'd really like is spaghetti and meatballs, just plain spaghetti and meatballs with nothing fancy added." She made him spaghetti and meatballs but—great cook that she was—probably added a pinch of one or another unusual spice. On the way home Al confided to me: "It was not quite right."

Dodie was on her way from Berlin to see Albert and she called from New York. He was happy to hear her voice but signed off a bit disconsolately: "I hope you get here in time." I took the phone from him and he went into his room to grade the last papers of the term. There was a crash and I heard him say: "Oh, God, what's happened to me now!"

What had happened was that he had landed on one hand and broken the skin. That promptly started an infection of cellulitis, which is a bacterial infection in the skin, excruciatingly painful and difficult to cure. The hand swelled and turned red; the doctor said to try to keep it elevated overnight and they would start antibiotics in the morning. That swollen painful hand, the first visible sign of Albert's mortal illness, became the focus for me of all the pity and sorrow that I had felt for months.

Albert was as direct with his oncologist as he always was with me and his friends. "How long have I got?"

"How long do you think you've got?"

"Not long. A few days."

"There's one thing we haven't tried. I haven't mentioned it because it's very experimental and also painful. Essentially it's a computerized method for focusing radiation very specifically on tumor sites. They take preliminary measurements in the morning and work with them mathematically all day. Then about dinnertime they radiate, briefly, what they believe are the correct sites. An unpleasant feature of the procedure is that you have to sit around all day wearing a kind of 'crown of thorns,' which is a metal band screwed at several points to your skull. This is so the coordinates are held constant. Sounds horrible, doesn't it? Do you think you want to try it?"

"If you were me, would you try it?"

"With this particular procedure, I don't know."

"What else is there?"

"Nothing."

"So I'll try it."

Tilly and I sat with him the whole day he wore the "crown of thorns." He bore it bravely, obviously feeling the strain of it but still able to joke.

The final radiation seemed to last a long time. The enthusiastic young technicians running around the machine and calling out readings irritated us. Mollie could not sit still but ran over and screamed: "You men there, isn't that long enough?"

It was an outpatient procedure and so we drove Albert home to bed. But Albert was gone. This last procedure had taken away his personality.

That night he and I slept alone in the house. I don't know how much he slept, though. Chairs were moved and doors opened and I heard movement. Around five a.m. he told me: "I think you'd better call an ambulance." He went out the door with the paramedics—on his own two feet and with a wry smile. He saluted me and knew I would get the reference. Several months ago we had seen the play *Tru* with Robert Morse as Truman Capote. The play ends with Capote walking cockily offstage to his own Last Exit—and saluting.

In the hospital elevator Albert started screaming. The oncologist and I had promised him he would never have any pain and, now that he had it, it was my name he screamed, feeling betrayed as well as tortured. While he was put to bed I ran from room to room, looking for the nurse who could order morphine.

"For God's sake, hurry up, that man is in agony."

"I'm moving as fast as I can. I had to help this young woman first. She's only twenty-four years old."

The implication that youth was more to be pitied than age infuriated me. But the morphine and the poor sick brain together put Albert into a coma. There began a week-long vigil, with some of his friends always there in the room or the hallway, but he did not speak at all and seemed to recognize no one. Mollie returned to New York and could not bear to come again unless Albert would recognize her. Dodie arrived too late to be spoken to. She brought with her a letter addressed to Albert, telling him all that he meant to her, and was convinced if she read it to him he would understand it, though he could not speak. She sat at the head of his bed and read softly while I sat holding his hand. I tried to believe that his finger twitches signalled comprehension. Dodie was sure they did and, of course, they may have done.

The hospital staff said there was no telling how long the coma might last and advised us all to go home each night. I am sorry I took that advice and feel remorseful that I followed their advice. The doctor called early one morning and said: "Professor Gilman has passed away."

Albert is buried in Mount Auburn Cemetery, where many well-known Cambridge writers and scholars are buried. He has one of the last plots in this beautiful old burial ground, and one day I will share it with him. Tilly had wanted him to be buried in New York City with the family, but I wanted him with me in Cambridge. Tilly's husband, Bernie, understood somewhat better than she what her sisterly devotion kept vague. "Tilly," he said, "they've lived together forty years, for heaven's sake!"

Albert listened to the discussion and settled it like Solomon: "Tilly has many people who love her. Roger has only me."

On the gravestone Albert has top billing. Not because he was first and my entry is not yet complete, but to make up for all the times he took the smaller bedroom and the lesser portion.

Chapter 2

Career Crisis

In the fall of 1989 Albert and I already knew Al's lung cancer had spread, but an announcement came from the San Francisco Opera that three cycles of Wagner's *Ring* would be performed in the summer of 1990.

The San Francisco Opera had done the same three years earlier and we had attended with our old friends since graduate student days, Marian and Joan Sanders, who now lived in San Francisco.

When we all left Ann Arbor back in 1953, as I mentioned, Joan had a nervous breakdown; Marian left the doctoral program at Michigan and took a teaching job to support the two of them. She found a good job in the California junior college system (no PhD required) and a pretty apartment in San Francisco and Joan found just the right job as a town clerk. When their lives were once again on an even keel, they wrote us with warm affection and suggested a reunion in San Francisco. Meeting again, we rediscovered why we had enjoyed one another so much in the Golden Duet days, and it became an annual thing for Al and myself to visit for a week each summer.

The 1986 *Ring* had been a big success. The performances were good and San Francisco used supertitles, which are essential if you are going to take any interest in Wotan's endless duets with Fricka and with Brünnhilde, not to mention Alberich or, even worse, Mime. The Sanders sisters, assiduous students always, boned up on the *Ring* and its characters and all the family connections before the performance and were entranced.

Albert and I decided to subscribe once again in 1989 to encourage the gods to keep Al alive, but it had not worked and in August I found myself in San Francisco alone. I went to the operas with Marian and Joan and invited one or another former student living in

San Francisco to use the ticket bought for Al. Daytimes and evenings I spent wandering the city.

I was staying at the Stanford Court at the top of Nob Hill, the most elegant hotel in the city, and I was not counting the cost. Here, as at the Ritz in Boston, I lavished money on room service as if I thought it could deliver something I needed. More accurately, I did it just to piss away money. Al had been so careful with money, expecting someday to enjoy it, only to leave it pointlessly behind in my hands.

Just two blocks down the hill, but very steep blocks, lay gay San Francisco. For me it was one big tease, in particular the Nob Hill Theatre. The Nob Hill is not just a pornographic movie house. It is a total sex emporium.

Inside the theatre there is an auditorium with a tiny stage and runway and a string of twinkling lights. It is here that the live, all-male, all-nude sex shows take place. These shows are not strip shows but jack-off shows. The young men start out naked, or nearly so, and to loud rock music, progress from penis play to erection and ejaculation. Or try to. A $20 ticket to the Nob Hill is good for the day. You can come and go as you like on the one ticket from 11:30 one morning until two o'clock the next, conceivably catching all five live shows. If you stay in the Nob Hill Theatre, there is a large collection of magazines and a large collection of videoboxes to study in an effort to read their relevance to your inner life. The possibility of making a contact is always on the agenda and becomes increasingly urgent as the day goes on and the blood becomes supersaturated with whatever chemical it is that makes men horny.

For me, on the day of which we speak, there was in fact no possibility at all of a contact. The Nob Hill is a lively place, but "who calls that livin' when no boy won't give in to a man what's lived sixty-six years?"

At 1:30 the projectionist announced a five-minute break in the movie to be followed by a personal appearance by talented young Kevin, porn star from LA, making his final guest appearance in San Francisco that very day.

Picking a seat in the cinema was a task calling for thought. It was not necessary to sit next to the runway to get a close view; the boys worked the whole auditorium. Starting at the runway, the performer in sneakers, athletic socks, and nothing else either walked up and down the aisles, or else mounted the arms of the chairs and, like Spiderman, picked his way overhead. In either case he might pause as long as he chose at any given client, thrusting his penis forward, or turning his butt around. It definitely was not important to sit close up.

It *was* important not to sit close to anyone else. Certainly you did not want to sit near some senior citizen who might try comradely knee contact. You might like to sit near one of the younger and more attractive men, but then he would be sure to move and that would hurt your feelings. Besides, there was a reason to sit apart from all the others: The performing boy was free to apportion his time as he chose. Some chose to stay away altogether from the more unsavory and to concentrate on just two or three clients. Only by sitting apart could you make such concentration possible and be sure that you were the intended target. This was important, because even though you knew the whole thing was a show for money, the mind somehow contrived to think of a disproportionate allocation of time as personal "attention," a singling out, a kind of compliment. Yes, even while you worked at creating the effect by stuffing dollar bills into the boy's socks.

The law allowed performers to be touched, but not on the genitals or buttocks. The information was broadcast before each show, and there were signs adding that the legs and stomach and nipples were all in bounds. But who could enforce these rules? Only the boy himself. The guy aiming the spotlight cannot tell what may be happening on the dark side of the moon, but the boy can feel it and permit it—or not.

"Gentlemen, please take your seats now and welcome our star, Kevin!" The applause was light, but, then, there were only eight spectators in the afternoon of a radiant day outdoors.

And there he was, his back to the audience, doing a kind of disco dance that made his little white buns jiggle. Turning to advance down the runway, Kevin was anointing himself with what I took to be oil, but then recognized as the brand-name lubricant "WET." Kevin wielded the lubricant as if it were an aphrodisiac charm, but he needed it as well to make slippery the pressure he was applying to his very pretty but totally uninvolved penis. As it stayed uninvolved, his massaging and pulling hand curved into a cup as if to shield it from scorn.

Kevin looked twenty-two years old. He was truly a boy, very nearly a skinny kid. Not tanned, not pumped up, not quite clean-shaven or well-barbered, but with a fine face suggesting intelligence and sensibility. He must have known that everything about him appealingly denied being the jack-off dancer he was trying to be.

Kevin tried to make it up to the guys with lewd postures and ingratiating smiles, but his anxiety was evident. Some brute got up and ostentatiously walked out. Kevin moved into the audience, thrusting desperately close and miming an arousal that his penis authoritatively denied. When he stood above me, dripping perspiration, I smiled up at him and said, "Take it easy, son; you're beautiful," and slipped a dollar bill into each sock.

Kevin smiled a real smile and said: "I like it when people talk to me."

I said: "You're not a machine; don't worry about it. You're too good for this crowd." I slipped him another buck and Kevin smiled and winked and we were alone together in our minds through the rest of the act.

Kevin never did get it up, and when the announcer realized he was not going to, he called out: "Thank you, Kevin. Let's hear it, gentlemen, for those beautiful buns." All that could be heard was one person, too loudly clapping. I abruptly stopped when I realized that the failure of my initiative made it more evident that Kevin had flopped.

Back home, before coming on vacation, I had read in *The Advocate* that San Francisco had come up with something new in commercial safe sex: "The Touchy-Feely Room." I planned to locate it and give it a try. Indeed, I planned to try everything, because when Al died I found that lust is a pretty good painkiller. You could not call it up every time you needed it, but for me it was a rousable monster about once a week. It is an ugly thing to say, but I thanked God for lust and hoped it would last as long as I did. In San Francisco, where Albert and I had gone almost every year for the forty years that we were together, there were many reminders that cut with a sharp edge, and I counted on the city's erotic inventiveness to subdue sorrow some of the time.

And where should the Touchy-Feely Room be? In the Nob Hill Theatre, of course. It was a bit embarrassing to ask "How does the

Touchy-Feely Room work?" but I managed. On one side there is a boy in a box–not quite a box, in fact, but a tiny room, a cubicle. On the other side, with a glass wall between, sits the client. You had to pay another ten dollars on top of general admission to place yourself in the client's seat. Molded into the glass wall, fingers in the boy's space, open wrists in the client's, were two immense elbow-length pink gloves. The client might handle the boy as he liked with his hands in the gloves, while a timer ticked off three minutes. The gloved hands could apprehend shape, size, and weight, but not texture or warmth. Condoms for the hands the gloves were, condoms as thick as inner tubes.

There is not a boy in the box at all times, but only as scheduled. Usually, the J/O dancer takes a turn after performing and Kevin nipped right in. I paid to be the client, and Kevin and I moved toward one another like reunited lovers.

"Is this a career crisis for you?"

Kevin started to laugh it off, but switched: "In a way, I guess. I don't like it when the audience is small and they just sit there looking grim. Anyway, I'm a student."

"I thought so. I'm a professor."

"Wow! A professor! That's what I hope for eventually. English lit."

"I want to buy your video to remember you by."

"I'll show you which one, but my picture's not on the box."

I did my best to hug him with my thick pink hands.

"I like it when you hold me," he sighed.

"That's because you feel the affection in it." Kevin put his hand on my hand. I said: "I like it when you touch me. It's you doing something, and not just me."

After some rapturous seconds I asked, "How come the timer's not gone off?"

"I didn't set it."

We stood and for almost a minute we kissed through the glass.

"I'll be back after dinner for your nine o'clock if I can get away in time," I said, and put twenty dollars in the tip box.

"You're a very sweet man," he said. "Handsome, too." My heart sang.

During the day Roger, faithful to Kevin in his heart, took in another J/O dancer who was more successful than Kevin had been.

The penile erection is a response controlled by the involuntary nervous system and so, as all men know, cannot be made to happen, as an arm is raised, by intent alone. The response is in fact impeded by anything like effort. But the second and successful J/O dancer had developed what you might call a "technology" for controlling the response.

He closed his eyes to the scene before him and concentrated on some fantasy that reliably turned him on. Erotic mental imagery is, as married folks know, responsive to volition and, if you can just keep your eyes on the inner screen, your body can often do what the situation requires. The dancer's face was all determination. His eyes were clamped shut; his brow was furrowed; his mouth was pursed and produced a faint whistle. One knew better than to speak to him. When at last he did ejaculate, his eyes popped open and he grinned at the audience, as pleased as if he had pitched a no-hitter.

All day my mind was on Kevin. I was determined to get away from dinner in time to see him again and that proved easy. My companion was a former graduate student, Tom Moore, on whom I had once had a crush. A crush is not reciprocal. After taking his doctorate, Tom had told me he was gay and we had had several pleasant reunions in recent years, recalling and reinterpreting the past; and I looked forward to telling Tom about my little adventure with Kevin. But Tom, a native born-San Franciscan, was bored with gay stuff and wanted to talk psychology.

"In my tutorial this week we read your paper on 'Flashbulb Memories' and it started a really good discussion."

I myself liked the paper, which was written in 1976 with Jim Kulik, one of the brightest students I had ever known. The prototypical flashbulb memory was the lively, almost perceptual memory everyone had for the circumstances in which they first heard of the assassination of President Kennedy. It was not the fact of the assassination that was special; it was the fact that people could recall the personal moment—what they were doing, where they were, who told them, and also idiosyncratic details which were accidentally in the focus of attention: "I was lighting up a Viceroy cigarette"; "I saw a terrified look on my teacher's face"; "I remember the feel of rubber tread on the stairs of Emerson Hall." As *Esquire* magazine put it in a feature story years after the event, "Nobody forgets": Julia Child was making *soupe de poisson;* Tony Randall was in the bathtub; Billy Graham was on the golf course but felt a presentiment of tragedy. "Flashbulb" seems an apt name for such memories because they are sudden, brief, bright, and long-lasting; it is not apt insofar as it suggests unselective registration of everything within the circle of light. The memories are selective in that only percepts above some threshold of attention are preserved.

I got the idea for the experiment when I noticed that absolutely everyone everywhere had a flashbulb tale to tell about the JFK assassination, whereas only my friendly bank teller, a black woman, told me a flashbulb story about the shooting of Martin Luther King—she was yelling at her son to come in from playing basketball when she heard. It occurred to me that flashbulb memory might be a special memory system fired only by events of high emotionality or personal consequentiality. The JFK case was perhaps unique because the handsome, idealistic young man had made the whole world kin. For every individual there might be individual flashbulbs created by highly personal emotional events, important news about one's own kin, and also flashbulbs shared with significant social groups: the slaying of black leaders for blacks, the letter of admission to Harvard for Harvard students, the first menstruation for women. With Jim Kulik, I had explored, in a famous paper, the idea that major news events, especially assassinations, created flashbulb memories in just those groups for which the events were most consequential or emotional.

"What my tutorial really loved," Tom said, "was the historical precedent. I read aloud quotations from Colgrove's 1893 paper on memories for Abraham Lincoln's assassination thirty years earlier. The parallels with the JFK case are amazing."

"I know, I do that too. But don't you find that students now tend to discount the whole flashbulb memory idea because of Ulric Neisser's persuasive counterexample?"

"You mean the business about his vivid but false flashbulb of hearing the news of Pearl Harbor the day before his thirteenth birthday while listening to the broadcast of a baseball game?"

"That's the one. And he says the memory was so clear that he did not question it for years, not, in fact, until our flashbulb memories paper. Then he realized its inherent absurdity. No one broadcasts baseball games in December! It was real but fake, essentially a fabrication or construction. My students find this anecdote more compelling than any systematic evidence."

"But haven't you heard, Roger, there's something new in the story." Tom wriggled with delight at what he had to impart. "There was recently a 'Note' in *Cognition* by Cowan and Thompson at Kansas State. It seems they heard a radio interview with Red Barber; you remember him—he's been a sports broadcaster for years. He was asked if he remembered the bombing of Pearl Harbor. And he said: 'Indeed I do.' "

At this point Tom took a photocopied page from his jacket and read:

" 'I was at the Polo Grounds to scout the New York Giants, who had already won the eastern division and were to play the Chicago Bears in two weeks for the championship. I was to broadcast that game. The Giants were playing the old NFL Dodgers. At halftime Lou Effrant of *The New York Times* came down from the pressbox and said Pearl Harbor had been bombed by Japan. I got up and went home. I was sick.' What do you think of that?"

I looked blank. "Don't you get it, Roger? This vindicates your assumption that flashbulb memories are real memories. That they are veridical. Neisser's recall was quite accurate rather than totally inaccurate. He was listening to a broadcast of the football teams who have the same names as two famous baseball teams. Furthermore, the game was played at the Polo Grounds, the home field of the New York Giants baseball team. I think we might say, 'Neisser was hoist by his own petard.' " And Tom glowed with pleasure at being the bearer of such good news. His glow dimmed a little when I looked unexcited.

"It's certainly a cute story and I am going to enjoy telling it." I checked my watch to see how near it was to nine o'clock. "The story is not all recall, though. In part it is a construction, and I guess we have always known that complex recall is both memory trace and construction."

Tom looked disappointed and I felt disappointed in myself. At one time an outcome so dramatic would have fired my imagination, would have initiated a flood of ideas about how construction related to memory traces. But not this evening. This evening psychology

did not seem to matter very much and the only memory I cared
about was Kevin. I hoped he was not going to have a career crisis of
his own. But nothing more was going to happen tonight, and the
time was 8:30, so I clapped Tom on the back and jumped in a cab to
go see my own sweet Kevin.

I had thought to arrive after the show started, imagining that,
having first missed me, Kevin would be glad to see me after all, and
that I might be an arresting figure in the dark with the light behind
me. But I could not get myself to tell the cabdriver to take me to the
notorious Nob Hill Theatre and could not remember the street
names, so I gave rather unspecific directions that landed me two
steep blocks away. When I got there I was so winded and panicky
that I had to sit down before the performance began.

Once again the audience was invited to welcome the evening's
star, Kevin from LA, and reminded of the rules of contact, and
assured that the performer welcomed tips. For this nine o'clock
show the audience was large, every seat taken. And there was Kevin
in the spotlight with his heart-stopping smile, once again splashing
himself with WET. But, dear God, there seemed once again to be
some question whether the performance would work.

Only then, when I saw that it was not going to work, did I realize
the risk of returning. I had imagined Kevin would be bound to
succeed and so it would be great to have his new friend there. I
really had just not thought of Kevin's *performance* at all, of the
likelihood that Kevin himself had been worrying about it all afternoon, and hoping not to see anyone who had witnessed the earlier
problem. I simply wanted to see Kevin and talk some more. But
Kevin was going to fail again, maybe even because my face brought
back in a flash the earlier panic.

I looked in every direction except Kevin's and Kevin at anyone
but me. The performance was ended, as the one in the afternoon had
been, at an arbitrary point, cut off by the announcer. There was no
applause at all.

Obviously now there could be no going back to the Touchy-Feely
Room. I left the theater and climbed the two steep blocks to the top
of Nob Hill to my hotel, where I dialed room service.

Chapter 3

Dream Boys

Dream Boys is Boston's most successful escort agency. "We offer you more than you get from your lawyer or accountant for the same hourly fee. Handsome, charming, built young men for the male clientele." The fee is $220 for one hour and a half. "Built" means possessed of a good-sized penis. An escort is not a dinner companion; an escort is a callboy.

And the ad tells the truth. These Dream Boys offer more than an attorney or psychiatrist–or just about anything else you can get for $220.

"Dream Boys" is a wonderful name for an escort agency because the boys are initially created from dreams. When you call, either Jonathan or Bruce will answer: "How may I help you?" Just "How may I help you?", which says nothing about the nature of the service and leaves it up to the client to know, which he will if he is "legitimate." If you ask about the boys available tonight or tomorrow you will be told a Christian name, perhaps "James," and be given a description: "James is 5'10" and weighs 160 pounds. He has deep blue eyes and chestnut-colored hair, cut very short. He has a completely smooth body. He has a swimmer's build." (Everybody who is not a bodybuilder is said to have a swimmer's build.) His shoe size is 8 1/2. "He is very versatile." (This means he tolerates some range of intimacies). "And he is very affectionate" (meaning he kissed someone once). The client's imagination goes to work on these few data points, and he soon has a fully fleshed-out image in his mind, an image he can summon.

When the image appears at the door it is bound to be surprising but rarely disappointing and always accurate with respect to the advance data. Dream Boys, the agency, interviews aspiring boys and inspects them before taking them on.

There are also instructions in self-presentation designed to correct anything that might clash with the modal dream of the clientele which is, above all, wholesomely boyish. No cologne ever; leave it to the clients to perfume their own flesh. No jewelry either; Jonathan has been known to say: "That earring will have to go." Reeboks on the feet, not too new and a little bit dirty; Jockey™ shorts impeccably clean. A fresh shower before setting out. Use the bathroom, having asked permission, before getting close. Quite a few of the boys, those from working-class families, ask: "Can I use the restroom?" which makes the place sound like a truck stop.

The first thing a boy on a date must do is "call in," letting Bruce or Jonathan know he has arrived on time and that everything is okay, that he has been met by one person, and not a posse of men and dogs. After one hour and a half the boy must again call in and will be asked: "Have you been taken care of?"–which means paid, and, if he has, will be told: "Then come on home"–which means head for the office in downtown Boston to hand over the $110 which is the agency's share.

Before sex, Dream Boys engage in conversation, which gives them an opportunity to be charming, as advertised. If offered a drink, they ask for a soft drink or "just water, please"; "no alcohol" is an agency rule. Then they will converse, easily, and yes, charmingly, but not necessarily truthfully, about their daytime jobs, their earlier lives, their career hopes, and remote dreams. "If my mom knew what I was doing right now. . ." How does he like working at the agency? "It's okay. It's interesting. The pay is good. No, nothing very bad has happened on a date." He does not expect to be doing it much longer.

The information given out on the first date is never very specific; it is generic in the way of the "fortunes" of a skilled fortune-teller. With Dream Boys on the first date the goal is always the same: Let the client construct his fantasy. Do not do or say anything that will disturb the process. Be his dream.

The transition from conversation to sex often threatens the dream. Of course the lead must be left to the client; that is simply good manners. With a Dream Boy on a date there is the additional consideration that what the client is "into," what "turns him on," must be made manifest if the boy is to realize his dream. But there's the rub. The boy may not be willing or even able to do what the client would like best. However, he must not deal the client a narcissistic wound by showing revulsion or incapacity but must gently guide the hands elsewhere, gently adjust the posture, or mime an approximation, a simulacrum. As Jonathan and Bruce have taught: A boy must know how to take control, and stay in control without overt conflict.

A client who cherishes his dream probably should never see any particular boy more than once. It is in conversations after the first that you get more boy and less dream. For lack of anything else to say he may start telling you personal truths. Perhaps he has a lover with whom he zestfully does all those things he has avoided with you. Or the boy's own erotic ideal, he may tell you, has qualities X, Y, and Z–which are not qualities you possess, and he will seem not to realize that this is painful news because surely the client knows that what they do together is strictly for money. Or–the boy does drugs, fails to wash, worships Barbra Streisand, or says "you and I" for "you and me." No, dreamers had best see a boy just once.

It is on the first date also that the sex is best. It is on this first date, if ever, that the boy gets hard and goes in for deep kissing. One wonders why. Perhaps strangeness or anonymity is simply an aphrodisiac. Perhaps it is just the wish to do a good job with a new client. Perhaps, however, the boy, like the client, has a fantasy, a dream . . . which is least disturbed, because information is minimal, on the first date. The boy, after all, determines how good the sex will be. It is the client who initiates, but the boy, as the gatekeeper, determines what will be permitted, and he is maximally permissive on the first date.

There is a boy (his agency name is Mark) who was hired while under a misapprehension about the clientele. To another Dream Boy he said: "I bet you meet some hot babes in this job." When he learned the truth he switched orientations without missing an appointment. We all have much to learn from the young.

* * *

When I first began seeing boys from Dream Boys, I was dying to talk about it with someone who would be interested in the social psychology of the encounters and not too shocked, and I chose

Leslie and Fabian, a female couple, who had long been dear friends to Albert and myself.

In fact they were shocked and outraged, in a political sort of way. They identified the boys with nineteenth-century working girls forced into prostitution and myself with some sort of capitalist pig, a conception that I thought off the mark.

"You don't understand the power relationship; the boys have most of the power."

"I don't see how. You have money and they don't," Fabian said, "and so they are forced to have sex with someone they would not ordinarily have sex with."

"But the money is not for the necessities of life. It is for the little extras, small luxuries. Many of the boys are students, not as many as say they are, but quite a few. And those who are not students have daytime jobs—waiting tables, for instance—and welcome the chance to earn some quick extra money."

"You don't know what may be a psychological necessity for these boys today. They could be as desperate for clothes and cars as women are to feed their families. And you certainly don't know whether they welcome the chance to be prostitutes. Just because this is not New York and you don't read about random bodies floating in the Charles doesn't mean this business isn't ugly."

I frowned. "The interesting thing is that the boys don't seem to find the work distasteful at all; they seem even to enjoy it. Yet here they are, in my case, with a man much too old for them, someone they would never look at in a bar. If I, for instance, approached one of them in ordinary circumstances, I would be dismissed with contempt. Yet as callboys they set out to charm me and respond with warmth and even sexual excitement. My theory is that putting sex in the service of entrepreneurial enterprise changes everything. When making out with an older man, or whatever kind of unlikely person, counts as a business success and not a loss of face it becomes satisfying in some way."

"My God, Roger dear," said Leslie. "What a comfortable self-serving theory. Men who use prostitutes always think like that. It's like . . . that it's a prostitute's art to give this impression."

"But Dream Boys, more than the women you are thinking of, really control what goes on. The only thing the client's money can accomplish–and I do admit it is something–is bring the boy to the door. When the boy sees the client, if he doesn't like his looks, he can reject him, using the excuse of not feeling well."

"And how often does that happen, given the power of the situation?" Leslie said.

"Not often. But it has happened. I know a boy who drove all the way up to Maine and, finding a half-drunk man and a house stinking of cigarette smoke, turned around and drove back without a word. But even though boys seldom reject clients, they reject acts. Frequently. They don't have to do anything they don't feel like doing, and they're all trained how to decline gracefully."

"Roger, answer me this. Do you think Albert, with his sensibilities, would have used Dream Boys?" Fabian said.

"No, but refusing ever to pay for sex is associated with having been very sexually active as a young man, and very, very successful–one of those people who are able to have anybody. This was true of Albert but not of me. Sex appeal and prowess were important to Albert's self-esteem. For me they are not; for me there is no ego in sex."

Fabian snorted. "There's something wrong with *that* formulation. All the time you've been talking about your Dream Boys it has been clearly gratifying to you that these twenty-year-olds find you appealing sexually and seem not to be reluctant to make love. They keep alive your image as a sort of Peter O'Toole, ravaged but still dashing." I recognized that this was exactly correct.

Leslie topped Fabian: "I don't like the feeling I get when you talk about this. It's not you. It's like cold stone. You think your theories are more important than these boys." I recognized there was also something in this.

* * *

While Albert never paid for sex and I did–many times–it was Al who introduced into our lives knowledge of how to *go about* buying sexual services. After Albert's death I recognized that what he did was an act of generosity, to provide me with information I would need, if I were to find any sort of sexual excitement in my later years–information I was too proud and too timorous to obtain for myself. This was in 1978, before AIDS, and it was some time before I made use of what I learned.

Al had a roguish colleague, Simon Smarm, a professor of French literature, fat and gross, whose only wit was sexual insinuation. This man, though married to a woman, knew all about the world of callboys. Al rather liked him. I could still afford to despise Simon and therefore did. Albert brought Simon home to teach us both how to make a phone call responding to an escort ad in the Boston *Phoenix*. Smarm taught by demonstration.

"Hello, is this Brian? Brian, my name is Simon. I'm responding to your ad in the *Phoenix*. Could you tell me about yourself? Yes, good. *Very* good, very impressive. Are you cut or uncut? How versatile are you? Would you say you are a bottom or a top? I see, it depends. Isn't that the truth? Well, frankly, I like to get fucked. Would that be a problem? Good. And what is your fee for an incall? I see, you only do outcalls. Well I live in Brookline. That's fair. So, Brian, I had tomorrow evening in mind, around seven, but I'll call to confirm."

I froze. This Simon with his gross belly and stubby, nicotine-stained fingers was a salacious brute. "Cut or uncut?" "Bottom or top?" "I like to get fucked." Never in a million years would I make such a phone call. About this, at least, I was correct. I would make many phone calls responding to escort ads, but I would never use indelicate language or ask crude questions.

Simon made several calls while Albert or I listened on the extension, and Simon explained why one response was more promising, more appealing, than another. "Peter is too cheap. The boys compare prices and there are no bargains. Peter would inevitably turn out to be substandard in some way. Kevin interests me. There was that touch of embarrassment that appeals to me. Not too experienced. Not too hardened."

Al and I did not pay too much attention to the comparison. The important thing we learned, and it sank in permanently, was that these calls could be made easily, routinely. The person responding knew what the caller wanted and was not at all perturbed. Expectations meshed and the whole transaction was quite ordinary.

On the day of Simon's demonstration, however, the language of the call, the look of Simon, and the nature of the bald exchange threatened me so severely that I was huffy to Simon and even cool to Al. Cool to Albert because Al had set up the event and therefore could be thought to have wanted it more than I. In my mind Al stood always under suspicion of betraying our relationship. When we had first met, I had pressed for a "faithful" relationship and claimed to be up to it, while Al refused even to try. This difference placed me on the higher moral ground which, against all the evidence, I had held ever since.

I could remember my first escort date better than most of those that followed. It was five years after Simon's demonstration, 1983, long before my prostate cancer and Albert's death. Gay men were terrified of the AIDS threat and very unsure about what kinds of sex were safe. They told one another jokes about the elaborate preparations now required for an act of love, something like a surgeon getting ready to go into the operating room. What I could never later recall was the dire necessity that drove me to try out the escort business for the first time in such an age of anxiety.

Simon's well-remembered demonstration made the phone call easy, but Simon had not explained how to do a close reading of advertising text, and a close reading would have spared me a bad beginning. The "boy" had not specified his age, and he looked to be in his late thirties. The ad had not claimed that Fred was handsome; he wasn't. He also did not look quite well; in fact, he looked *sick*. He was effeminate, too. And sarcastic in a nasty way.

I had plenty of time to take in all the unappetizing facts before anything got started because the ad required me to phone from the public telephone on Massachusetts Avenue and Beacon Street and wait to be picked up, standing under the streetlight so that I might be inspected in advance. I passed Fred's inspection and we walked three blocks to Fred's apartment, with me saying to myself the whole time: "I can't go through with this. I can't possibly go through with this." And yet I did, which shows that Leslie was right about the power of the situation.

Fred's basement apartment was revolting: soiled sheets on a couch and three long-haired cats with Kitty Litter and plates of soured milk all around. "Payment in advance." Fred held out his hand and smirked, then everything happened very fast. Fred snapped on a porno film at a preselected scene which made me think: "My God, look what they are doing!" I was pushed back on the couch, my penis pulled out and snapped up by what felt like a rubber mouse trap. I ejaculated instantly and then saw Fred tossing into the corner a used condom. The experience put me off callboys for the better part of a week.

The next date was much better; another basement incall but a boy with a handsome face and a tanned muscular body. I ejaculated twice and the boy, Scott, professed to be envious of such capacity.

I saw Scott soon again and thought: It's really wonderful that for a sum of money that means very little to me I can enjoy such a good-looking boy. And to some extent my appreciation was transmuted into sentiment. Scott had asked me to send a postcard from San Francisco when Albert and I went there to see Marian and Joan. Al happened to read the postcard, and, noticing that it hinted at feelings, said: "Another betrayal, which doesn't surprise me."

Back home again, I called Scott right away and was disappointed to be put off for three days because "My mom is visiting me." Disappointed, but understanding and sympathetic. The poor kid, supporting himself in a way that would kill his mom if she knew. How guilty he must feel and how worried that something would give him away, an unanticipated phone call, failure to clean something up or put something away. I willingly cooperated by not calling, and, at the end of the three days, when I went to keep our appointment, I was prepared to discuss seriously with Scott possible changes in his lifestyle that would make him more respectable without excluding me.

Scott did not recognize me or remember an appointment; he stood in his underwear, glassy-eyed, not shaved, and stinking. The apartment was torn up; the toilet unflushed. Looking into a closet I saw leather gear, ropes, and chains. Without fully understanding, because I lacked the background, I could see that something frightening to me had been going on. Scott's "mom" had been some kind of sadomasochistic leatherman, or whatever, and Scott seemed unlikely to be interested in a more respectable lifestyle. From these early encounters I learned, not chastity, but that agencies are better than individuals, outcalls better than incalls.

* * *

As a result of my prostate cancer surgery I was left sometimes, unpredictably impotent. But I was a big man who had always been "good in bed" and, while the doctors I saw all seemed to assume I would just retire my sexuality, I did nothing of the kind.

When a man loses his prostate he loses the ability to ejaculate. Impotence means the inability, occasional or permanent, to achieve erection. Impotence is not a necessary consequence of prostatectomy; loss of the possibility of creating semen is. Impotence is listed as a low-possibility risk on the form one signs, giving permission to operate, and I had given it with almost no thought in advance. The infernal twist is that desire and the possibility of orgasm are not removed even though the possibility of satisfying desire and achieving orgasm would seem to be.

Would seem to be, but actually are not–not quite. Desire is of the brain–not the prostate–and so is orgasm, assuming the possibility of some minimal friction. Desire is somewhat time-dependent, becoming easier to arouse with the time elapsed since the most recent orgasm–even as it is in the intact specimen. For me, in my mid-sixties, it usually took about a week, and what can an orgasm be when there is neither ejaculate nor full erection? Certainly it is not what it used to be. There are spasms and, afterwards, something of the nervous relaxation and abatement of desire that follows normal orgasm. It is, all in all, a state worth striving for, though just barely.

My prostate cancer was followed in only a few short months by Al's vastly more terrible lung cancer and an operation that left him looking like something in a meat locker. When I looked at Al's upper body I felt my heart bleed. They say your heart does not literally bleed, but it does.

The operation was successful and Albert and I started out in June on our tour of the Far East almost unworried about health. In Japan Al began to have trouble keeping his balance and then trouble walking. Amazingly, no doctor had told us that when lung cancer metastasizes the most likely site is the brain.

Months later, when Al was dying, pictures taken by a member of the tour group were sent, and there was one of the entire group at a luau, or some damn fool thing, early in the trip, everybody smiling and a little high on beer except, dead center, Al was staring out at the camera, his eyes wild with terror.

In November of 1989, when he had only about a month left, Albert delivered a summing-up of sex. For forty years Al and I, like many couples, had been fighting over sex. I hated Al's compulsive cruising. Al didn't know the meaning of love, or how to express affection. No, Roger was the greater sinner because his infidelities were emotional, even when not physical. Al was incapable of emotional infidelity because Al was incapable of Love. Et cetera, et cetera. Many times I threw together a few clothes and toilet articles and stormed out at night "forever," only to crawl back in a few hours.

"Sex," Al said in his summing-up. "Since I've been sick I've not thought of sex even once. So much for sex, the distinguished thing."

After the funeral there were many months of sorrow and remorse. What gave relief were the exigencies of teaching two seminars of twenty students and a required paper each week. Forty papers to read and grade plus two class preparations kept my mind mostly in the present rather than in forty years with Al. When the term ended and I made my first attempt to stay in the Braithwaites' house in Provincetown, which I had rented for the month of June, things were quite otherwise.

"Is there an escort service in Provincetown?" This to a young lesbian cabbie who had picked me up at the airport.

"No, there isn't, and I don't know why not. We certainly need one."

Calling Dream Boys long distance, I arranged to have a boy drive out that night all the way from Boston. Not for sex, really, but just to have something human happening. The boy turned out to be someone I had seen before and not liked much. I had not recognized either the name or the description; I might have recognized the description if it had included the one most memorable feature—bad teeth—but of course it had not. The boy, naturally enough, thought I remembered him and asked for him and so I had to hide my disappointment and be lively and pleased, which was trying and dreary. The next day I fled Provincetown, its isolation and memories, to get back to Cambridge, where I had a routine and people to telephone and a kind of emotional room service.

* * *

Later that summer, and in the academic year of 1990-91, I saw a callboy almost every week. When school was on, Friday was special, not only for the end of the work week, but because the Boston *Phoenix*, the paper in which callboys advertised, came out. Most of the time I called the agencies, either Dream Boys or its short-lived competitor, Jason, but I studied the individual ads to see if there was anything interesting that did not fit the agency molds. Acting on one of these almost always turned out to be a mistake: Dream Boys and Jason exercised quality control and there was a level of appeal below which their boys never fell. Individual operators, on the other hand, were chancy. Not that they blatantly lied, but you had to read very carefully indeed. If something relevant was left unspecified–age, weight and height, "looks," penis, versatility–you would be sure to find the escort disappointing–possibly grotesque–in that one respect. And because I was adventurous and sometimes careless, I met in this way several overweight or overaged gentlemen. On the other hand, I also met "two hot college jocks, together or alone." Their names were Gennaro and Tony, and I had them together since the agencies did not offer this toothsome possibility.

Twosomes that advertise are generally partners or former lovers. If you get together with such a pair, you must expect to find that their anxiety about sustaining the relationship in some degree constrains what can happen with you. In Palm Beach two years later I met a handsome pair, Nick and Sean, whose unspoken compact was to hold inviolate the top and the bottom of the digestive tract or, operationally, no kissing and no fucking. Between Gennaro and Tony there was also an understanding of some kind, but it was subtle and emotional, not topographic.

Gennaro and Tony complemented one another both temperamentally and physically, and so, it seems, do all such pairs. Gennaro was the bold one, the foreign secretary, the one who answered the telephone and talked terms and counted the fee. He also took the lead socially. One time after the three of us had had a very good conversation on an abstract philosophical topic, I asked: "Now how do we make the transition to sex? How do we segue into the bedroom?"

Tony, knowing his partner, said: "Leave it to him; he can always do it." And Gennaro could.

The subdued member of a twosome seems also to be the one who feels more keenly the threat of the business arrangement to the marriage. In the case of Sean and Nick, I ventured this observation: "Nick is the more sensitive one, the one who is more uneasy about your threesomes." They allowed that this was true. And just to make mischief I tried to hand the fee to Nick, who looked at it wonderingly until Sean stepped forward to grab it. For the team of Gennaro and Tony, the sensitive one was Tony.

The physical complementarity of twosomes is as striking as the temperamental and a major selling point. Sean, on the telephone, described himself as a serious bodybuilder with impressive "abs" and "pecs" and then, quite sweetly and with some awe: "Nick is handsome." Gennaro had a smooth, white "bubble" butt. Tony was tall, dark, hairy-chested—a Montgomery Clift look-alike. One wonders how the complementarities of temperament and physique come about. Perhaps they are one another's biotypes and perhaps biotypes tend to be complementary. Or, perhaps, one day it just dawns on pairs of this type that, taken together, they comprise an ideal lover, with something to please everyone, and they decide to make of themselves a single package.

Tony and Gennaro told me they were both former students at Yale, Tony a graduate student of philosophy and Gennaro an undergraduate in a section led by Tony, and I believed them. They were able to converse on a level of abstraction not common in such encounters. What on earth did these two students and a professor, these two boys and a man, find to do in a sexual line? Something between a dormitory romp and a wrestling match, with both friendliness and sensuality in it.

Once Tony said: "What shall we call this, a sandwich?" and thereafter they both said "Let's make a Roger sandwich! Or—a Big Bob burger." Once, when the three of us were wrapped together into a monkeyball, I in a kind of epiphany, said: "Isn't it great to be together in this way? We could be teachers and students in the ordinary way and never get close like this."

Then I did something for the first time that I was to do many times, with increasing extremity: I tried to expand the client-callboy relationship, expand it into something that would fill more of the empty spaces in my life. I invited Tony and Gennaro to fly with me to Provincetown and spend a weekend at the Braithwaites' house. There was plenty of space; they two could sleep together in the big bed in the master bedroom or apart in any of three smaller bedrooms. Of course I would pay all expenses. Gennaro looked interested but Tony held back.

"Of course you would be losing income, and so I would want to give you something extra for your time."

"I don't like that aspect," Tony said. "We would be your guests and yet taking money like employees."

"That could be worked out," Gennaro said. "It's true that we could hardly afford to take the whole weekend off without pay, but it obviously could be much less than our usual hourly rate."

Tony said: "We would just take the weekend off if this were an ordinary invitation from a friend."

"Tone', we don't have to decide now. Let's you and I talk about it. It's a very nice invitation."

I went on: "I know it's a little bit unusual and awkward but our whole friendship is highly original. All we need is goodwill and a little imagination. You're probably wondering if you'd be expected to spend all your time with me. Definitely not. For one thing my bedtime is ten and I'm sure you stay out later than that. None of my friends keep the hours I do. We'd all just do what's comfortable."

And there the matter rested for two weeks. I had golden fantasies about the weekend with the two sweet guys who had melded in my mind into one sweet guy, an object of tender desire. The fantasies were all dreams of arrival or departure. They all took place in the tiny Cape airplane: feelings of high anticipation taking off early Friday morning or else weary, contented camaraderie flying into the golden sunset Sunday evening. My mind seemed not to dwell on what happened in between.

The weekend never came to pass. Presumably because Tony and Gennaro could not resolve the dilemma: what was I to them—client or friend? This time it was Tony, the sensitive one, who did the talking on the telephone. "I couldn't take money from you when I was your guest. And what would we do each evening? Come in and kiss you good night at ten and then go out on the town? Thank you for inviting us, but it wouldn't work."

"I understand," I answered. "I'm disappointed, but I understand." Recognition of the impasse made it impossible for me to call anymore. Six months later I noticed that their ad had disappeared from the *Phoenix*.

* * *

My adventures with Dream Boys seemed to me so interesting that I badly wanted to talk about them, but not any more with Leslie and Fabian. Not with any women. With a man, a gay man, a gay man interested in psychology who had some experiences of his own to disclose. The rest of humanity was too loaded with "attitude" to do me any good, or so I thought. Jack Quilty, my best friend, seemed the likeliest candidate, and I had several times come close to telling Jack what I had been up to and then stopped because it seemed to me that the picture was just too unsavory—a man in his sixties, with my handicap, carrying on in such a fashion.

Jack had once been my student, but that was ten years ago. Now he was a full professor at MIT in the field of personality and abnormal psychology. I thought him the most brilliant person in the field and also the most sensitively nuanced reader of character, what Freud called a *menschenkenner*. He was also a compassionate person. If someone in a group was hurting, Jack was the first to know it, and he would be there with some kind of healing balm, saying or doing whatever would help. When he said something that made me feel good, and he did that all the time, I would tease him: "I can't tell whether you believe this or you're promoting my mental health again."

There was one big mystery about Jack—his sex life. His friends and colleagues did not know his sexual preference, and everyone was interested because Jack, in addition to his brilliant mind and sweet nature, was a good-looking man of the buttoned-down Cambridge type.

People supposed that I, as Jack's best friend, must surely know something about his love life, at least whether Jack was heterosexual or homosexual, but, for several years, I knew nothing. Jack would talk about going to parties or to Harvard football games, and would use the pronoun "we," and I would ask: "You and who else?" and the answer would turn out to be some married couple or social group—an answer totally opaque with respect to the information sought.

As a graduate student, Jack had, for one year, shared an apartment with my student in San Francisco, Tom Moore, and when I lectured there in 1987 Tom and I had dinner, and I asked the question that puzzled academic Cambridge: "What's the story on Jack Quilty? Is he one of them or one of us?"

"Amazingly enough, I don't know. I think he's just asexual—some kind of Peter Pan innocent."

"There is no such thing."

"Well, then, maybe he's bisexual. He always had both male and female friends, but he never spoke of any of them in sexual terms, and I never saw any physical intimacy."

Jack and I became best friends because we enjoyed one another's minds, had the same wicked sense of humor, and were both, in a secondary way, literary men. My apartment building was right at the edge of the MIT campus, and Jack fell into the pleasant habit of stopping by late Friday afternoon for a drink or two and good talk.

In spite of my warm feelings for Jack, I felt no sexual attraction. That is the way it is with gay men: friendship excludes sex; they are different musical keys. Indeed, when a gay man falls in love and so must play in both keys, he very often has potency problems. Jack was also never attracted to me. Possibly, I thought, because Jack is not gay, but even if he is the age difference would rule me out.

At some point in the friendship, and I could not pinpoint when or how it happened, I came to know for sure that Jack's sexual preference was the same as my own. It was not because Jack said so or because he ever referred to any homosexual actions of his own. It was just that he understood too perfectly and too quickly my allusions and presuppositions. And so, without any acknowledgment either way, it came to be taken for granted.

The knowledge that both were homosexual deepened the sympathy between Jack and me, but knowledge is not the same as acknowledgment. For two men who loved conversation as Jack and I did, the difference was great. I longed to share Dream Boys with Jack, to talk about his theories and hear what Jack thought of them, to enjoy the play of Jack's insight and ironic intelligence on the new subject, but, for a long time, I could not come clean. This was because Jack himself seemed so wholesome, so much the shirt-and-tie straight guy who did not even swear or use obscenities. I could not comfortably contemplate the contrast with myself unmasked, myself in the altogether. And then something happened that made it easy.

Our good friend Tom Moore got in trouble at Minnesota before he went to San Francisco for sexually molesting a male student and was fired over it. "I don't know why he did anything so foolish," I said, "when there are fairly safe ways to meet young men."

"And what ways are these?" Jack asked. "I'm interested."

I described the way that Dream Boys operated, and confessed to my own involvement. Jack's reaction was exactly what I hoped for. High interest untainted with morality, an almost anthropological curiosity plus a still-cautious personal inquisitiveness. Then, finally made trusting by my potentially embarrassing self-disclosure, Jack began to talk about himself.

"The main thing to understand about me is that I am not grown up. I can read people well, especially the agendas they don't know they have, and I have some small talent for personality theory, but I myself, in my private life, am not grown up. Our friendship is the greatest intimacy I have known."

"You must be kidding—everyone's crazy about you."

"I was in my prime at Harvard College. Harvard men and women don't talk about their achievements, of course; the place is too competitive for that. Instead you complain about the yoke you share: impossible reading lists and having to write six papers in two days and nights. For the list of achievements, you have to read the personal résumé. They are always impressive but mine—you are the only person I could say this to—may have been unsurpassed in my year. I hugged this thought to my heart as a student and I'm still hugging it."

"I know you were a *summa*. A Harvard *summa* is one of life's few real distinctions."

"I did graduate *summa,* and my honors thesis won a Hoopes Prize. I also wrote the Hasty Pudding Show in my year and was president of WHRB and barely missed getting a Rhodes. These things helped, but it was my roommates who really made the times wonderful. Three great guys. And I was the center of our shared hours."

"What does that mean?"

"They thought I was basically the same as them but a little smarter or more mature. Each one confided in me as in no one else. They used to joke that I had psychic powers. And I did know how to make fun. I organized groups to go to games or just for pizza takeout for the four of us. We talked about our parents, about the future, about sex and women. We walked around in our underwear."

"Did you know you were gay?"

"I knew it–always, I think–but my roommates didn't. Not that anyone ever made jokes about faggots. Even then it was not politically correct at Harvard to admit to any prejudice against homosexuality. Nothing anyone did sexually could shock us–that was our group position. Whatever gets you off. The one thing we couldn't stand was effeminacy, camp, acting like a ponce. But that was a matter of personal style unrelated to sex and we had a right to our preferences in this area. And I took care, as a leader must, to overconform–to be the most masculine of all."

"What a drag!"

"And I'm still doing it–successfully, I think."

"Very successfully. So successfully that you must be putting off all the men who may be interested in you. But do you really want to do that? You're forty and spending your time taking care of your mother and escorting women to meaningless dinner parties. You're missing out on sex and intimacy and even authenticity. It's getting late. This is not just a dress rehearsal, you know."

"I know it! God, don't I know it! Like Antonio in *Merchant*–'the blasted wether of the flock,' that's me. But that long love affair with my straight roommates ruined me. I can't stand any effeminacy, anything campy. I guess that makes me homophobic these days, but it isn't political, just a personal turnoff."

"Jack, if you want to try Dream Boys, you can specify 'very straight' and they will deliver."

"It seems safe enough."

Between ourselves Jack and I started referring to Dream Boys as "d.b.s." "Are you free tonight or do you have a d.b.?" A d.b. took priority over anything else, we both understood. It was our little code, signifying a uniquely close understanding. For both, composing a report of the encounter and theorizing about it came to be more fun than most encounters.

Jack did not see nearly as many d.b.s as I did. One of his alternatives was calling an occasional number in the "Men for Men" personals in the *Phoenix*; the kind that begins: "BUSY DOCTOR, 35, handsome, straight-looking and acting, has no time for bars, games, phony people. . . ." Mostly it was a complete waste of time, but Jack did meet one bisexual man who taught him something new about himself.

"What did he teach you?" I asked.

"It's something very personal. Hard to say. He got me to try something I had never tried before. People never think of it for big men like me. But I liked it, that is I. . . ."

"You don't mean you liked taking it up the wazoo? You like getting fucked? I should have guessed, but you're so fastidious. It's true that people don't think of it for big guys like you, but it's often just the ticket."

"I don't know that I'd say it's just the ticket, but in any case I'm seeing him every two weeks; I think he's more heterosexual than bisexual."

* * *

While Jack saw only a few d.b.s, because they were not very satisfying for him, it was Jack who brought into our lives the most interesting d.b. of all: Michael Broad. It was characteristic of Jack that Michael, the only dream boy who ever satisfied a dream of his, satisfied a dream of personal sympathy, not sex.

As related by Jack to Roger, the first meeting with Michael went something like the duet "O namenlose Freude" from *Fidelio*, in which Leonore and her long-imprisoned husband Florestan sing of the inexpressible joy of reunion. Jack and Michael were soulmates, identical twins separated at birth, now breathlessly discovering identities and affinities.

"You're from Louisiana? But I'm from Louisiana?" "Not Shreveport? Me too." "You write poetry? So do I." "Who's your favorite songwriter?" Both together: "Cole Porter." "What's your favorite play?" "*Antony and Cleopatra*, of course!" Now almost screaming: "Your father committed *suicide?* But my father committed *suicide.*" Then, really screaming: "Let's do it. Let's fall in love. Camels do it. Sheiks do it. Nice young men who sell antiques do it. Let's do it. Let's fall in love." After all the excitement sex could only be an anticlimax. And it was.

"What does Michael look like?"

"He looks like James Dean. James Dean in his prime, and you can't beat that. He says he's a Phi Beta from Duke. He certainly has the intelligence and cultivation."

"Why is he working as a d.b.?"

"Just for the hell of it, for kicks. He used to have fantasies about it and so he decided to act them out. He doesn't need the money because his family are immensely rich and they send him a check every six months. Between ourselves, Roger, I think he's being a d.b. as a kind of revenge on his mother. He sees her as a whore on a large scale because she married his father for money."

"He really sounds interesting. I'm looking forward to meeting him."

Jack brought Michael the next Friday afternoon and I, of course, instantly fell for him and grew envious of Jack, whose good looks could enable him to interest James Dean. Michael had brought a tape, on Jack's urging, of himself singing songs he had written. Michael, as he listened, closed his eyes and made an intent face; Jack did the same, even more intent; I felt like giggling at the lyrics and gagging at the tunes but kept silent. At the end Jack said (and would be kidded about this forever), "Those songs are brilliant; they are touched with genius." Michael said: "You really think so?" I kept my counsel.

Then Jack, in order to give me a chance to shine, said: "Roger loves opera and knows more about it than anyone."

"I love opera," said Michael, surprising the other two.

Uh oh, I thought, now he's going to try the natural affinities routine on me, the O namenlose Freude bit. The little phoney. No one his age with his looks loves opera. Then aloud: "Really? Which operas are your favorites?" To myself: It's going to be something learned from the movies–probably *La Boheme* out of *Moonstruck*.

"Bellini is my particular favorite."

You had to give him credit. He knew some surprising things.

"Which Bellini in particular?"

"*I Puritani.*"

I thought I would pass out. My own favorite! The very title, I would have said, known only to opera queens and musicologists. There must be some profound natural affinity between myself and this boy. Something deeper by far than anything Jack and Michael might share. Excited by the opportunity to play my best cards in a rivalry over love, I said: "Let me show you my record collection!"

To my surprise, despite the great size of my record collection, Michael clearly preferred Jack to myself, probably because Jack was twenty years younger, better looking, more fun, and always able to get it up. This lack of discernment caused me to wax both jealous and envious and generally ill-tempered. It did not help that Jack in his kind way tried to keep me from feeling left out. That was the way I nevertheless did feel. Especially when they called, all high spirits and jokes from the nearby Sonesta Hotel—the same room.

"He probably thinks we're fucking our brains out" was Michael's canny diagnosis. I *had* thought that, but felt only marginally better when Jack told me the two had tried sex just the one time and were not likely to ever make another attempt. "The trouble is," I thought, "they are so close to one another, so much closer to one another than either is to me."

Michael was not making enough money with Dream Boys to meet his expenses. This was only a temporary embarrassment, of course, since his check from home was due to arrive soon, but in the meantime he was short of cash. He was fed up with Dream Boys in any case because Jonathan and Bruce were deliberately not sending him out on many calls. "I know I'm popular, probably the most popular, but those two madams don't like me. They think I'm a smart-ass because I won't toe their stupid line."

"Why don't you cut yourself free of the agency?" Jack suggested. "Set up as an independent. You and I and Roger can write the best ad the *Phoenix* has ever carried."

Michael liked the idea, and the two of them, with no help from me (I was sulking), wrote an ad that was indeed very successful.

> James Dean
> Blond, blue-eyed, innocent
> Does it all

In November Jack caught the flu and it got worse and worse and stayed with him for weeks. His doctor wanted him in the hospital but Jack would not give up his privacy and all the things he loved in his Harbor Towers apartment: the computers, the music system, the exercise apparatus. The Towers was a wonderfully dramatic building, looking out to the open sea with buttresses like outflung welcoming arms. Jack could not bear to leave for a bed in the hospital. For a week he staggered around the apartment, heating up TV dinners and calling his office many times a day, but he could not manage shopping for food, laundry, the library, and the post office, and he got blue being so sick, all alone.

Michael started doing Jack's chores, adding one to another, until he was a general factotum. He let many of his outcalls go by in order to do Jack's errands and was happy doing it because this meant more of Jack's company, which he so enjoyed. Jack insisted on paying him, and Michael insisted that the pay be small.

"Michael, why don't you move in here? I mean, if you wouldn't mind. You'd have your own suite, and it would save you money. I've hesitated to ask, because clearly it would be wonderful for me."

"Me too, you big dope. I'll make meals and clean up the place and be a real little homemaker—and nurse. The first thing I'm going to do is put an intercom on the phones so you can call me at night."

" 'Let's do it. Let's fall in love. Scallops in their shells do it. They say that even Orson Welles do it. Let's do it. Let's fall in love.' We'll get a new phone line for your outcalls and when you're out on errands for me I'll take messages for you."

It was in this way that Professor Jack Quilty of the Massachusetts Institute of Technology came to operate a callboy service out of his home.

Then Matt arrived. Matt was Michael's long-time lover from back home in Shreveport. He was a touch handsomer than even starry Michael, and, on Michael's testimony, the number one lover in the world. Matt moved in. And these two, in Jack's apartment, but with the doors closed (and quietly), did fuck their brains out.

I imagined that, in this situation, Jack surely must be jealous. Al had once said to me and Jack: "I don't really like *Othello*, or rather I don't understand it because I have never experienced jealousy." I had been incredulous, but Jack had chimed in: "I'm the same. I've never cared what anyone was doing with anyone." I was well acquainted with the green-eyed monster and had never understood that Jack and Michael were pals, buddies, and that sex entered into it almost not at all. But pals they were and Jack was not jealous.

Michael knew how I was, knew that I was not capable of being a pal to a beautiful boy. Michael may have worried that I, early on at least, might try to avail myself of a citizen's right in a free society and so call Michael's number and book him. Whether Michael ever thought of that possibility, he decisively closed it off by telling Jack, in my presence, what he would do if someone absolutely unacceptable were ever to call: "I'm sorry, you have the wrong number. This is the AIDS Action Committee. There's no James Dean here."

For just two days, Michael, with Jack's help, hid from Matt the nature of the business he was in. Each time the phone rang Michael, or Jack, would sing out: "I'll get it; it's probably for me." But one time they were too slow and Matt heard: "Is this James Dean?" Matt, who was well aware of the resemblance, said he was and so heard: "I'm responding to your ad in the *Phoenix*."

Matt managed to be horrified for two whole days. He really could not be too horrified, because he himself had often thought of selling his body, and then there was silver-tongued Michael assuring him that it was the most harmless thing in the world, fun to do, and a great kindness to others. It was no threat to the love Michael bore Matt, because there was no emotion in seeing a client. It was a kind of gymnastics, probably good exercise. Come to think of it, why didn't Matt try it? He would see for himself. Michael bet Matt would be more popular than Michael.

Matt did try and he was.

Do not try to imagine Jack's state of mind. I could not. You had to be Jack. He was having a marvelous time. Remember that the calls were all outcalls; horny men were not ringing the doorbell in the middle of the night. And the two merry callboys had wonderful stories to tell.

There was the Trampoline Man who taught at Christian Brotherhood College in upstate New York and drove to Boston to have a pretty boy bounce on his great belly for an hour or so. Michael said he didn't mind but wished he could bring a book. There was the time a call interrupted Matt's push-ups and, as he headed for the door, Jack asked: "Aren't you going to shower? What if he wants to lick your armpit?" Matt laughed: "I'll tell him it's not on the menu tonight."

For Jack, this was a return to dormitory days in college, a return in which all the boys were handsome and clean. Speaking wistfully at a later time Jack said to me: "And you know, around the apartment both Matt and Michael were gentlemen. They never walked around naked. They didn't think belching was funny. They closed doors on private functions. Their main occupation, hours at a time every day, was grooming. They were two beautiful, wholesome, housebroken hairless anthropoids, and I shall never see their like again."

Matt had concentrated in psychology at Louisiana State University and, for about twenty-four hours, he and Michael thought they might settle down in Boston and Matt would do graduate work in psychology at Harvard. I, of course, was expected to get him into Harvard but, as yet, Matt and I had not met, and so a dinner date was set for the three of us plus Jack.

In the afternoon, by way of preparation, Michael showed Matt my most recent book. Matt read a few pages from the chapter on human sexual behavior before dozing off. Michael took Matt to the reference library, pulled down the current *Who's Who in America*, and had Matt read the long entry under my name.

I was very much looking forward to the dinner. From Jack I had heard what a glorious specimen Matt was and I planned to play my full deck of Harvard cards: condescending a little but warmly encouraging, flirting with the possibility of admission to graduate work and whether that could be managed. When we met, greatly to my chagrin, despite the great length of my entry in *Who's Who*, Matt clearly preferred Michael and Jack. Probably just because they were younger, better looking, more fun, and always able to get it up–the same reasons Michael had preferred Jack to me.

Jack recovered from the flu and started spending most of the day at MIT, but Michael and Matt stayed on–not because Jack needed the help but because he was so happy having them with him. At Christmas he felt he would have to have a minimal, two-day visit back home in Shreveport with his mother's family. Matt too would be going home; both his parents were living and they doted on their handsome son. Only Michael and I had nowhere to go for Christmas, no one back home we wanted to see, certainly, but also no one who cared about seeing us. That made us the lucky ones in Jack's eyes. Still, Jack knew, even the most alienated person could feel a bit hollow alone on Christmas Eve. He fretted over his two orphans and finally suggested to me that, both being opera lovers, Michael and I spend Christmas Eve together in my apartment, listening to music and getting to know one another.

The suggestion suited me. Despite Jack's unremitting efforts to include me in his happy family, the family was really complete without me and I felt more isolated than I had when Jack and I had been two against the world. But what I most wished for just now was not Jack but Michael, who was as attractive to me as ever, an intimacy founded in the subterranean bond whose only surface manifestation was the incredible shared appreciation of *I Puritani*. A cozy Christmas Eve over opera might provide the opportunity to, in harsh terms, cut Jack out–and Matt as well.

Michael had never shown any interest in digging up the roots of the *Puritani* phenomenon and, indeed, since his initial dazzling success in answering my Opera Quiz, seemed rather to avoid the subject. There were indications also that my appearance was unappealing to him, even repellent. He had once said to me, "Your hair is nice; it's your best feature," which did not sound like much of a basis for intimacy. However, the Christmas Eve proposal clearly meant a lot to Jack, who wanted the two friends to be as dear to one another as each was to him. So Michael went along.

I thought a lot about the musical program for the evening. It could not be any ordinary, generally available CD or video, not for a *Puritani* fancier. I had in the past two years discovered a new natural affinity, an affinity amazingly enough for a twentieth-century composer: Leoš Janáček. It had been a great thrill to discover that Janáček's masterpiece *Jenufa* moved me almost as much as the masterpieces of Verdi, Wagner, Puccini, and Strauss. Therefore, I unconsciously reasoned, I was not the hopelessly regressive nineteenth-century sentimentalist that some people thought, but a connoisseur able to recognize and be moved by true genius of any era. Recently I had obtained by mail order a videotape of Janáček's *The Makropoulos Case*, featuring as the 350-year-old Emilia Marty, Anja Silja, who used to be, as everyone knew, the mistress of Wieland Wagner.

The Makropoulos Case should be the evening's entertainment. It was a little risky because Janáček's music was not made up of ravishing long-lined melodies in the nineteenth-century style but of short-breathed melodic fragments that took a little getting used to. But how exciting it would be if Michael, like myself, discovered in this superficially unpromising stuff the glorious expressiveness of the nineteenth-century masters. Discovery of a newly shared natural affinity ought to be emotionally, perhaps even physically, overwhelming.

Michael had been shopping at Tower Records, getting some new heavy metal and country and western and also something to prepare him for Christmas Eve with me. He dropped his acquisitions on Jack's couch and went to get his mail. I was waiting for Jack to come in with their drinks and, passing the time, looked over Michael's purchases. And what to my wondering eyes should appear but "Puccini's Greatest Hits" and "Opera Without Words."

"Michael? Hi, this is Roger. How are you? Michael, I've been thinking about Christmas and feeling rather blue about happy memories of past years. And Michael, I hope you don't mind, but I think I had better spend Christmas Eve alone. It's nothing serious, but I would just be very poor company."

"I can understand that."

"We can have our opera evening another time."

"Sure, any time."

After New Year's, quite suddenly, with little advance discussion, Michael and Matt were gone. They had spoken vaguely for some time of going to San Francisco, but Jack had not realized this was a real plan until he came home on January 5 to find a note saying they were on their way, with a postscript longer than the note telling him how to feed and care for the cat—their cat. The cat crying, arching its back and rubbing up against his leg, sharpened Jack's feeling of abandonment and he felt like flinging the cat out into the ocean. Instead, he called the woman two flights down, whose little girl always made a fuss over the beast, to ask whether they might not like to have it for their own.

Jack and I resumed our Friday afternoon chats. Jack would call around five and say something like: "I'm tired of normal people. Can I come over and talk dirty with you?" We didn't really talk dirty; neither one would have been any good at it. We talked honestly, ironically, theoretically about the mysteries of sex and love. One of the major mysteries to both of us was Michael. Who was he? Was he really a Phi Beta Kappa at Duke? Was he really rich? Did he really love poetry? There were very many pieces of evidence that argued, especially to Jack, that Michael was exactly what he claimed to be, but there were also fragments that did not fit. A letter from Michael to Jack came on February 3. It answered all the questions.

Dear Jack:

This letter comes to you from Dallas County Jail where I am. The police claimed that Matt and me stole three million dollars in jewlry and tryed to fence it in London, N.Y.C., Dallas, et cetera. We should be so lucky? If true we'd have money—right?—and we don't have any. Hopefully, our lawyer will get us off but I don't know, they say they have the goods. I might get a 2-year sentense. Matt is not even here with me. They nabbed him in San Francisco.

Anyway Jack I just want to let you know what happened so you wouldn't think I just ran off without a thot for you. One thing I always admire is brains and you have that in spades. The Dallas police may get in touch with you to ask about me. All I told them is that I used to do errands for you and didn't ever steal anything and you treated me like a prince. Say hello for me to Professor Brown.

Yours faithfully
Michael

One week later Jack did get a call from the Dallas public defender, and, in time, he wrote what amounted to a glowing character reference. Two months later Michael wrote that he had been given a two-year sentence, but Jack was not to worry. Michael was very popular in prison and soon would be running things. He looked forward to seeing Jack and Roger in two years' time. As did Matt.

Chapter 4

Face-Lift

What I really wanted in the spring of 1991 was a lift. Something that promised to rescue the future from the list of inexorable changes for the worse. A face-lift is not something to do, exactly; it's something to undergo, a temporary retreat, a period of seclusion—deliberately becoming a chrysalis in order to emerge a butterfly. It is not surprising, therefore, that the face-lift plan was made at Easter.

I was in New York to see *Parsifal* at the Met. *Parsifal* in the spring had become a regular thing with the Met because of the feeling of hope and resurrection that is in the music. I had always felt this affinity between the season and the opera, and going to see *Parsifal* at Easter was a way of bringing into sharp focus the feelings of the season.

Like the season, the music is generative as well as sublime, and sometimes one quality gets in the way of another. As a boy I first experienced *Parsifal* from standing room at the Met, and standing room at the Met used to be, and probably still is, a notorious cruising spot. Just as the Grail was being unveiled for the final time, I felt an unmistakably carnal thrust from the rear and said: "Can't you, for Christ's sake, wait?"

Wagner's music is like that. Filled with yearning or *Sehnsucht* which is sublimated as long as the music is playing, when the music stops the excitement continues, possibly blowing off as cheers and applause but sometimes turning into what must in candor be called lust. Albert and I in our pilgrimages to Bayreuth never saw this, but we had heard it said that after a performance, the bushes in front of the *Festspielhaus* were alive with frenzied young satyrs working off the effects of the music.

The most satisfying Good Friday I held in memory was in 1984. It was warm and sunny but Albert and I groped our way into the cavernous, dank, and almost-empty Exeter Street Theatre to see Hans-Jürgen Syberberg's surreal film *Parsifal*. When we stumbled out, five hours later, the sun was setting but still bright enough to make us squint.

We had dinner at a crummy Chinese restaurant in Harvard Square and then went to see the Harvard Gilbert and Sullivan Players' *Trial by Jury*. Everyone on stage and almost everyone in the audience was fresh of face and brightly smiling. The boy who played the defendant recognized the two professors and winked at them as he sang:

> I smoke like a furnace,
> I'm always in liquor,
> I am such a very bad lot.

It was a good day, a marathon of music, a day of unforgettable intimacy.

Now alone, in 1991 *Parsifal* failed to work its spell. Not because of the performance, which was good enough. In fact, in 1991 the Met put on a new production of *Parsifal*. In the old production a scattering of crepe paper anemones had been counted on to suggest Wagner's fragrant green meadow. In the new production, it was anemones again, but mounted on individual springs which went "boing" every time Kundry or Gurnemanz or Parsifal stepped on one. The sound was gravely antagonistic to the effects of repentance for which the singers strove. But never mind, I thought, and closed my eyes to hear the rapture in the music.

But I could not find the rapture. I could only hear the sounds of musical instruments and voices. Now loud, then soft. How sad that the music which I had known since I was in high school should, now when I most needed it, have lost its potency.

I had thought of having a face-lift before 1990. What for? Not to look younger. Not to please Albert, who, in fact, did not like the idea. Just to look pleasanter, really, for the sake of my students and anyone who had to come close up. In recent years, I thought I had come to look rather sour, and that is what I sought to change.

Five years earlier, I had gone so far as to get recommendations from the Society of Constructive and Reconstructive Surgeons and, from *New York* magazine, had taken down the name of someone said to be among the best: Dr. Matthew Slyce. Dr. Slyce had told me: "You are a good candidate for a face-lift," but I had not gone ahead with it, perhaps because of Al's opposition, perhaps because I used to have better things to do. But now, why not?

The reason for having the operation in New York was that it would be difficult to keep it secret in Boston. Why should it be necessary to keep it secret? Good question. Cosmetic surgery, especially a face-lift, is not gender-neutral. It is something women go in for and men do not. That is an exaggeration, I knew, and somewhere I had read that more and more men, these days, are getting face-lifts. Even if that is so, the operation is still a feminine thing to do, though not exclusively female. The thought was not enough to deter me. I was fairly unconcerned about masculinity; at least I was in the Harvard-Cambridge milieu, where gender marking was not taken very seriously and no one expected me to set the high-water mark.

The more serious deterrent is what might be called "personal values." Whether the patient is male or female, the person who gets a face-lift is, by definition, superficial. Philosophers do not get face-lifts, nor saints. A professor of psychology, though not held to so high a standard, would still like to be thought sufficiently concerned with the inner nature of things to scorn a face-lift.

If the operation were to be in Boston, I could picture myself returning to the apartment, head swathed in bandages, like Claude Rains in *The Invisible Man*, and questioned by the security guard, the old ladies in the lobby waiting for the mail, and one or another Puerto Rican janitor. None of these interrogators would be shy about asking personal questions and none would be satisfied with inexact answers. In the healing period after the bandages came off, everyone in the damn building would scrutinize my face and manage somehow to suggest that I had wasted my money. No, thanks.

Staying at the Hotel Pierre in New York, it occurred to me that I could pop in there after the surgery and recuperate for a week or so, with room service the perfect solicitous and discreet companion. Why not take the shuttle to New York right after school in late May, have the operation before I could begin to worry about it, and then hole up in the luxurious Pierre, concentrating my thoughts on healing? When I could show my face again, it would be on the shuttle to Boston and, without even leaving the airport, board Cape Air for the puddle-jump to Provincetown, where I could stay in the Braithe-waites' house, already rented for June. It was right on the ocean and there I could swim and sun my scars away for the entire month. It actually sounded like fun.

"You will not be able to go directly from surgery to the hotel," Dr. Slyce said. "It is necessary to spend one night in the hospital because of the possibility of excessive bleeding. In New York one night in the hospital costs $3,000, which is not covered by Blue Cross and must be paid in advance."

Dr. Slyce was a tiny, perfect man with delicate hands, pink nails, and a face so white one felt it had never been exposed to the sun, an unspoken reproach to my orangish weather-beaten mug. Not that Dr. Slyce, for all his perfection of the newborn, was in any way appealing. Looks like a slug, I thought.

"You were a good candidate for a face-lift five years ago and you are a better one today. I have an open date on May 28 and we can do it then, but you must make a definite decision and pay a deposit three weeks in advance. My fee is $10,000. You must also see my colleague, Dr. Robert Snipp, within the next two weeks, because your eyelids should be done at the same time as the face-lift, and he does that procedure. Miss Glaze, here, who is my nurse, will give you the details."

Odd that Miss Glaze should be a nurse. She looked like a movie star or a model. The entire suite of offices seemed too glamorous to have anything to do with medicine. But Miss Glaze proved very serious, not to say insistent, even suspicious, when she took my medical history and asked for the list of medications I was presently taking. Probably in New York you learned that most people had something to hide.

I was not entirely candid about the number of aspirins and Advils and Voltarens I popped all day and several times a night to ease my arthritis and incidental fears and anxieties. Anti-inflammatories all, they were also blood thinners and would have to be completely stopped before surgery until ten days after. Cold turkey! I supposed I could do it. Also no alcohol for two days before and two days after. The face-lift started to look like not so much fun.

Back in Cambridge, Jack Quilty had a better idea. Jack was, among other things, a consultant on the staff of the Massachusetts

General Hospital. Mass General had on its staff one of the world's great plastic surgeons, Dr. John Kaswell.

"He does all the stars. I think he did Joan Kennedy. He's planning to retire from surgery in September but I think I can get you in before that. I'll call Sally Wussie, his secretary, and tell her how famous you are—show her the *Harvard Magazine* profile."

Other things equal, Boston made more sense than New York, but what about the problem of secrecy? Jack, in his way that recognized no flaws in his own grand schemes, had a dozen answers, all of them no good. He imagined, for instance, that I might speak in confidence to Ahmed, the security guard usually on duty in the evenings, and a good friend, and enlist his aid in the following way.

I should tell Ahmed that I had to have removed from my nose a skin cancer that was not at all serious. But I was embarrassed about the operation because my own foolish vanity would seem to have made it necessary. My neighbors in the apartment building had sometimes seen me on the roof sunning myself among the clothes-lines. One or two had even taken it upon themselves to chide: "Better not overdo the sun, Professor."

An operation on the nose would hardly account for a box of bandages encasing the whole head. You could forget that scheme, like all Jack's schemes.

The solution occurred to Roger himself: Don't go to the apartment. Substitute the Boston Ritz-Carlton for the Pierre. Stay as long as I was seriously unsightly and tell my friends that I would be in San Francisco—which had often been the case in late May and early June.

Jack had done a good job on Miss Wussie. She seemed thrilled to meet Professor Brown. Dr. Kaswell, a celebrity himself, was not thrilled but he was respectful to someone of a station comparable to his own. He was an elegant English gentleman, wearing a floppy yellow bow tie that was absolutely theatrical. He had what I had come to think of as a swashbuckling style, the kind of offhand audacity that characterizes a number of Boston physicians who are known as "tops in their fields." Whether the audacity came from exceptional success, or the success from the audacity to dare what lesser physicians feared to try, no one can judge.

"I think I can make you look a bit better." All the time Kaswell talked, a younger, shorter, apprentice doctor standing at his elbow paid close attention.

"Of course your skin has been severely sun-damaged."

"I know, but I don't really regret it; I've enjoyed the sun all my life."

"I understand; I like the sun myself, but it can be dangerous."

"Every six months I see my dermatologist, Dr. Basil Sell, and have him look me over for melanoma. Dr. Sell is wonderful. He knows there's no use telling me to stay out of the sun and so, when I turn up, he just exclaims: 'What a wonderful suntan!'"

"Really? That's almost malpractice."

"Dr. Sell isn't like other dermatologists. He's kind of a buccaneer. When Rogaine first came on the market for baldness, the *Boston Globe* interviewed lots of dermatologists and every one made a pussyfooting statement about the need for further research. Dr. Sell just said: 'What the hell! Try it!'"

"That's Basil Sell all right, and I suppose I'm a bit that way myself. Well, if you want to have the operation, I think I have an open date sometime in late May. What's the schedule look like, Sally?"

"May 23 is fine."

"That's perfect."

Dr. Kaswell said, "I'll have to do the forehead as well as the face if you're to look all of a piece. I'll lift the skin here to raise your brow about one-quarter of an inch and pin down the flap back here where your hair will hide it. There will be stitches along here and scars for six to nine months, so you'll want to wear your hair longer than usual. Otherwise the scars will be behind your ears, where no one will see—except, perhaps, your barber, just at first. I'll suction some fat out of your neck and tighten up your jawline."

"Sounds horrible, but I'm game. How long will I be in the hospital?"

"Oh, you won't. It's not necessary. In fact, they wouldn't take you; the operation isn't that serious. You'll need someone to take you home and to stay overnight. So, if you'll just let me take a snapshot as you are now. . . . There, that's settled."

In the outer office Miss Wussie filled me in on the details. "There will be a lot of swelling at first, and black and blue around the eyes, like a raccoon, and so you'll want to stay out of sight for a while. The bandages will come off after four days and the stitches will come out a week after that. In three to four weeks you'll be completely comfortable in public. So, if you follow your plan to spend June in Provincetown, that should work out perfectly. No one will see any dramatic change. People will just say you look rested, as if you'd had a long vacation."

As it turned out, no one ever did tell me I looked rested.

"How long will I have to stay out of the sun?"

"Only as long as the black and blue lasts, and that should be three weeks at most."

"What's the reason for staying out of the sun? Is it really necessary?"

"It's just that when your skin is bruised it's sensitive. You don't want to get a burn."

But, I thought to myself, I never sunburn.

And finally, "What's Dr. Kaswell's fee?"

"Forty-five hundred dollars."

"But that's very cheap. In New York a face-lift costs $10,000."

"Yes. Dr. Kaswell's fees are very reasonable." Her tone suggested that the great surgeon was not in it for the money.

Then came the medical history, medication questions, allergies, and so on. All answered in full except for one thing: Minocin, of which I took two large capsules every day of my life. Minocin, like tetracycline, prevents acne. It really works. I took it as an elderly adult, because I still stood in danger of the occasional zit. Especially when feeling the strain of an impending public performance. A trivial thing, really, but I thought what a lifesaver tetracycline and Minocin would have been for me and all adolescents forty years ago.

Dr. Kaswell, I reasoned, would not have more than a very approximate knowledge of Minocin. He might recognize it as a cycline and know about cyclines and sunburn and so direct me to stop medication and stay out of the sun. The beautiful, powerful June sun in Provincetown, so healing to the spirit. I judged that I alone could weigh all the factors and saw no reason to put myself at risk of an ill-informed medical edict which, if pronounced, I would not dare to disobey.

In all ways the Boston option was more attractive than New York. I would need someone to take me from the hospital to the hotel and stay overnight. Jack Quilty, as usual, was not at a loss for an answer: "We'll ask Paul." Paul was a librarian at MIT whom I had met several times. Intelligent, gentle, and a little bit humpy.

"Paul will be perfect; he is naturally compassionate and could use a little money. Take two adjoining rooms at the Ritz, and Paul can be there with you all night. I can come in the evening and we'll have dinner in your room. It'll be a lark."

Paul thought so too. It sounded like something out of *Auntie Mame*. I called on Kathy Johnson, who was in charge of reservations at the Ritz. "My name is Roger Brown. I am a professor of psychology at Harvard. On May 27 I am going to have a face-lift and I want to hide out at the Ritz afterwards."

In unflappable Ritz style, Miss Johnson said, "Of course. How may we help?" They would be happy to preregister Paul and me and spirit the invisible man through the lobby. "And, I hope your, ah, surgery goes well."

To my secretary, my students, my friends, I would be leaving for San Francisco on May 23 and would be there all through June. The morning of May 23 found me, however, on an operating table in Mass General—under local anesthetic.

Dr. Kaswell explained to his apprentice and I overheard: "The most difficult thing is raising the brow, because, you see, you have to cut some bone away."

SKRUNCH! It felt—and sounded—as if they were operating with tin snips. No actual pain, of course, until that evening at the Ritz. Offered Tylenol, I screamed for Demerol. Jack and Paul noisily dined on lobster bisque, Dover sole, and crème brûlée. The waiter expressed the hope that Professor Brown, in his blood-soaked bandages, would feel better in the morning.

The day the bandages came off I held my hands before my face and peeled away the fingers one at a time so as to take the impact—whether Jekyll or Hyde—area by area. The black and blue around the eyes did indeed make a raccoon mask—but that, I knew, would go away. The line of stitches at the hairline reminded me of Frankenstein's monster, and that line would be visible for months, but easily hidden by my forelock, which I need only neglect to slick back.

There was a red incision under the chin, but you had to look for it. There were swellings in all sorts of places. But behind all the marks of battery, I could see a noble conception: a firm jawline, a tight neck, a smooth forehead. A face, not exactly younger, but pleasanter, more serene, more approachable.

"You are brilliant! You have done a brilliant job!"

"Well, perhaps you will look a bit better."

"You look wonderful," sighed Miss Wussie.

And now I truly relaxed. For the first time in years, it seemed, I had no urgent academic project. For students and secretary, friends and acquaintances, I was out of reach, my whereabouts in fact unknown. And the worst of my mourning for Albert seemed to be lifting. I had nothing to do but heal. And each day would be brightened by the prospect of improvement, so long as the marks of trauma gradually passed away.

I found it very agreeable to take an early morning walk in the neighborhood. The Ritz fronts on the Public Garden, which in May is planted in tulips. Commonwealth Avenue runs along one side and in May, as I could see from my window, the magnolias and horse chestnuts blossom. On the other side is Newbury Street, where the fanciest shops are found: Boston's Worth Avenue or Rodeo Drive, but not so harsh.

Just one block from the hotel, across the street from Brooks Brothers, stood a huge square building, occupying a full block with its grounds. This had formerly been Bergdorf Goodman's and now was Louis, a most expensive clothing store. Louis, in his munificence, had placed inviting benches with backs on them on either side of the front lawn. I found it marvelously agreeable in the cool of the morning to sit for a few moments on one of the benches and feel the sun warm one side of my face and then to move to the bench opposite and warm the other. It was too early in the day for the sun to burn and, in any case, its rays fell only briefly on my face. Once or twice I sat down at noon at the outdoor cafe behind Louis and had a goat-cheese-on-croissant sandwich–but always wearing sunglasses and with sun shield on the areas of black-and-blue not covered by the glasses.

My walking habit was to go the length of Newbury Street in one direction and then to come back on Commonwealth. On Commonwealth there are benches beneath the great shade trees, and I would break my walk every few blocks to rest. The benches were well shaded except for a dappled light that broke through the leaves and I, heliotrope that I was, sometimes turned my face up toward the filtered light.

In my room, reading, I explored with my fingers the new face and scalp. The top of my head and the right side of my face were almost totally anesthetic. It would take six months for the nerves to regenerate. Under the hair, where the skin flap from my forehead was fastened, I felt what seemed to the fingers to be staples. And staples is just what they were, something I learned when they were later pulled out with pliers.

The strangest sensations came from behind my ears. My fingers discovered and obsessively caressed what felt like mossy patches. I told Jack and Paul: "I seem to have pussy behind my ears." It was, I discovered, my own beard pulled up by the face-lift. "You'll have to shave behind your ears from now on," Paul said. "Better get an electric razor."

One June 6 a male nurse, gay but pleasantly masculine, took out all the staples and stitches. "You're all set for another sixty years. Let me see the 'before' picture. Wow, that's impressive!"

"You look wonderful," sighed Miss Wussie.

"The black-and-blue hasn't faded at all yet," said I.

"Don't worry, it will."

That same day, June 6, I drove down to Provincetown to the Braithwaites' house, rented for the month of June. This would be the second summer I had it. And this time I thought I would be able to stay most of the month. I had first seen it in February of 1990, two months after Albert's death, and I had needed something to look forward to–as I had needed the face-lift this year. And June in Provincetown had looked promising. To have a house in June, especially a house on the water, it was necessary to act in February. My memory of myself on that freezing day in February, so like the day of the funeral, was that I had felt like Roosevelt at Yalta: weighed down, trembly, not up to the business at hand.

The house was just at the edge of town where the highway divides into Commercial and Bradford streets. The house had a big white porch, beach roses, and a pine deck with a ladder into the water. On the first floor the windows of the kitchen and dining area looked out on the bay, and on the second floor were two large bedrooms and eight large windows with the same view.

In June of 1990 I had made two attempts to stay in the house but each time had left after a single night. I had not foreseen how the town would scream of the past. With nothing to do all day, I was at its mercy. The past was not simply recalled: it was reconstructed and experienced as Albert, dying, must have experienced it. Our last June week there, in 1989, must have been less than golden for him, and I fled back to Cambridge to escape my remorse. This year would be different.

"I've had a face-lift," I told Susan and Pat, the lesbian realtors. "Only ten days ago. The black-and-blue will go away. In general, I'm enthusiastic about it."

"Great!" said Susan. "Now you'll do the whole bit and get the hair dyed and start life over. It's a great idea."

"No, just the face-lift. I like my hair okay. I didn't do it to meet someone. That's impossible; I'm sixty years old" (actually I was sixty-six) "and I'm only attracted to young guys, very handsome ones. I couldn't be interested in anyone my own age. I got the face-lift for my students."

I left out a disability that I thought disqualified me from any sort of erotic life: The operation for prostate cancer in 1988 had left me frequently impotent.

"Never say never," said cheery Susan. "You're a stunning man and from many points of view a catch." I smiled doubtfully.

The first weekend, Jack flew out to stay overnight, and I drove to the tiny airport in the dunes to meet him. Jack was happy to have this brief escape from his work and ailing mother. The two of us in the car felt free and exuberant. I turned on Callas screaming out Puccini's "In questa reggia" and opened the sunroof so that all of Provincetown might hear:

> *Gli enigmi sono tre.*
> *La morte e una*

"Louder, Maria, louder! Dead thirty years and more alive than ever!" It was wonderful to impose her on still sleeping P-town and to feel the morning breeze and sun on our faces.

Saturday Jack and I went to dinner with two couples, George and Steve, Alex and David. Pillars of monogamy to gay men in Boston, each couple had been together and "faithful" for about ten years. The two couples were necessary to one another as demonstrating that a real marriage is possible. "I don't know what we would do without George and Steve," David once said.

The dinner would be my first public exposure since the face-lift, and, looking in the mirror, I judged that they would be less likely to say "How rested you look" than "What on earth happened?" Should I tell or try to keep the secret?

Jack begged me to keep the secret. It was our thing, a bond of intimacy, the secret of best friends.

"I'm not ashamed. I'll just tell the—"

"Why don't you wait? They may not notice a thing."

Before dinner, the light not too bright, and sitting apart, no one noticed anything. Jack, vastly enjoying this company, so rare for him and yet so deeply congenial, was very funny and very diverting. But at dinner, with the circle gathered close under a strong light, I was sure I saw puzzled glances being exchanged.

"I haven't been in California: I had a face-lift and holed up at the Ritz. Tell the truth—you noticed the black-and-blue, didn't you?"

Alex said: "At first I didn't, but when we moved to the table I was horrified. I thought, what's wrong with Roger?"

David said: "When I was standing over you I saw the huge scar on your scalp and thought, oh God, you'd had brain surgery."

From the confession I learned not to fear coming clean, not to close friends who never thought me a paragon of either manliness or philosophical depth and were more pleased than not to discover a sign of any vitality at all. The face-lift made a pretty good story, especially the part about Demerol and Dover sole at the Ritz. Eventually I came to enjoy telling it—in strictest confidence—to each of my best female friends and on the occasion of my Fourth-of-July party in 1991. Each knew and each thought herself the sole trusted confidante until they began to make single trusted confidantes of one another. Then, three women betrayed, they turned on me like Donna Anna, Donna Elvira, and Zerlina advancing on Don Giovanni.

At the P-town dinner party the story of the face-lift occasioned dismay because it demonstrated that Roger, Albert's mourning widow or widower, and the symbol of the longest-lasting gay union anyone had ever heard of, had not been fully understood, would, in fact, have to be drastically reconsidered.

And then I was alone. Being alone in Provincetown had in earlier years been a deep pleasure. Several times in Albert's lifetime I had taken such a solitary week. I might speak to no one at all during the entire time. The day would be spent in walking, swimming, and sunning into a state of exhaustion, which came on about four. Then I would return to my small rented apartment, have a hot bath, and succumb to the sweetest sleep of my lifetime, a delicious nap with the sound of bees in the beach roses just outside the window.

Alone again now, the possibility of deep pleasure was gone. The deep security of knowing I would return to Albert was gone. The physical strength for daylong strenuous exercise was gone. Untroubled surrender to the sun was forbidden. And the narcissistic pleasure of seeing myself beautified by the sun was replaced by the horror of the raccoon mask which, on most days, seemed not at all improved as the extreme limit of three weeks approached.

"On most days" is right because my assessment of how bad I looked was very dependent on the mirror, the lighting, my mood, and even the time of day. From much scrutiny I discovered that after a night's sleep the blood did not fully return to my face until 12:30 p.m. Early in the morning, when my face was bloodless, the black-and-blue appeared as a fine sifting of soot just beneath my skin. I could not figure out why it should take this form. I had been told that as the bruises healed they would turn first green and then yellow, and I could see that this was true of a bruise on my leg caused by a blow. But the disfiguring mask on my face remained always the same shade of black.

When four weeks had passed after the operation, I had a panic and called Sally Wussie. I would have done so earlier but I knew that Dr. Kaswell was away until September.

"Sally, it's four weeks now and I don't think there has been any improvement at all. Does this mean something has gone wrong? Has it ever *not* gone away?"

"I'm not sure, but I'll ask the residents and call you back."

"I'd really appreciate it, Sally. I don't mean to be a nuisance, but this thing is really getting to me."

Sally called back in just a few hours, and I was deeply grateful. "The residents all say that it will definitely go away. We do remember now one woman whose bruises did not entirely disappear for about eight weeks. So don't worry about it. Yours have probably improved more than you realize and they should go away completely in the next few weeks."

"Oh God, thank you, Sally, and thanks for calling back right away. As long as they will go away eventually. Being alone like I am here, I start imagining terrible possibilities."

I made a quick trip to Cambridge five days later and, passing a mirror in the airport, a new mirror for me, quickly checked my reflection to find that Sally's prediction was, thank God, coming true. I saw almost no discoloration and, on my way out of town, I checked again; it was really true. Immensely relieved, I arrived back in the Provincetown house in a kind of paradoxical mood. After so much anguish, I felt that the problem need not end so precipitately. I had prepared myself for a longer wait; to have it all over in a trice seemed to mock the anxiety I had felt. Checking my face in the standard mirror at the house, the mirror to which my memories were calibrated, my heart briefly stopped. There was absolutely no change! A new mirror in a new light at a new distance had deceived me.

In August Dr. Kaswell returned to the office for two days and I flew in to see him. Miss Wussie saw me first. "You don't look bad at all! I thought I was going to see big black circles."

"In this light maybe, but there is a dark shadow around my eyes and down the side of my face that was not there before the operation. I know it!"

Dr. Kaswell led me to the examining room, turned on a powerful fluorescent light, came up close, and for several moments peered at my face. Then, incredibly: "What is it exactly that bothers you?" I mutely and from memory traced the perfectly clear boundary separating clear skin from discolored skin.

"I don't see anything that worries me." I barely refrained from saying: "Is that because it's me and not you?"

"You must remember, Professor Brown, that the color of one's face is made up of thousands of variously tinted bits of pigment, and your pigmentation is especially varied because of your being naughty about the sun."

"I know all that, but I'm not imagining things. Please just follow my fingers and you will see a contour separating a clear central area from a shadowed area under the eyes and on both sides. The contour corresponds to the original black-and-blue area."

"Hmmm. Well, there may be some slight . . . if there is, it's barely visible and may be expected to fade. I'll bet none of your friends has commented on it."

"Of course they haven't, but that doesn't mean they don't see it. They're considering my feelings." In my mind, but not aloud, I wrapped up the doctor's position as "There's nothing there and it will go away." The whole thing painfully reminded me of the position taken by the urological surgeon on the side effects of the prostate operation. Impotence was normal for several months but 99 percent of the time it went away. The urologist repeated this litany month after month and refused to be worried about the fact that it did not entirely go away.

I see how it works, I thought. They tell you that whatever it is either does not exist or will certainly go away, and so time passes, and so the patient lives with the disability and eventually habituates to it. The feelings of panic and outrage diminish and eventually life goes on—but at a lower level of adaptation. Habituation must be something they teach them about at medical school. And the most terrible thing about habituation, as well as the most wonderful, is that human beings can habituate to *anything*. People can, for Christ's sake, habituate to being quadriplegic. And all I had to do was habituate to a raccoon mask.

Albert, who would have been opposed to the face-lift, would have said: "You now look just the same except—you have rings around your eyes."

In the mornings of my acne years, I had needed a long time before the bathroom mirror in which to operate, lance, lotionize, and, in hopeless cases, apply a Band-Aid. The worst time had been in the Navy at Asbury Park, New Jersey, where I shared a converted hotel room with five lusty, large-boned, healthy young men from the South who had to shit, shower, and shave, all in about fifteen minutes after reveille. I remembered comforting myself with the thought that if things got any worse I could always jump out of the window, fifteen stories up.

One blessed spring in my twenties I discovered the cosmetic effects of sunburn. When the whole face is reddish-brown, then those reddish-brown spots that arise from internal toxins are less salient. I vaguely noticed that in the spring the sun brought remission, whereas midsummer seemed to exacerbate the condition; I had stupidly failed to formulate the principle that a little sun is good but a lot is bad. Instead I became ferociously and forever addicted to sunbathing.

In my parents' backyard, lying on an old bedspread with clothesline overhead, I took the sun. In Cambridge, on the little balcony of the apartment, which received effective sun only from eleven to twelve in the morning, I used a reflector of the kind you used to see around the necks of old people on Coney Island in March or October. Once, when an assistant professor, I laid myself out on a table and opened a big window in order to catch some rays in a small office I had presumed to be locked, and the departmental secretary had walked in on me. We had both been as startled as if taken in flagrante delicto and never after spoke of it. On tour in the Valley of the Kings, while the guide talked, I turned my eyes away from antiquity, in order to expose my face to the life-threatening, life-renewing Egyptian sun. At learned conferences and in classes, however interesting and important the subject, if the sun shone outdoors I chafed. I came to feel that any sun that shone, if it shone not on me, was wasted.

In sum, I had for more than forty years an addiction of almost unimaginable extremity and irrationality. Once in a bitter quarrel Albert had screamed: "You and your damn sun! On cloudy weekends I used to pray that the sun would come out so that I could be spared your bad moods." Not even Albert knew the full extremity of it, not even my psychiatrist. There are some things too crazy to confess to anyone.

The addiction ought long since to have killed me. I had supposed that it would—but resigned to it rather than moved to change. But it hadn't killed me. Instead it seemed still—to my own eyes—to improve my appearance. And I loved the feel of it; I loved surrendering to the sun's caress. It was as a precaution that cost me nothing in lost sunshine, and somewhat calmed the sense that I must die of it, that brought me to Dr. Sell for a semiannual inspection for melanoma.

And so in the month of June when the sun is most welcome, and also the strongest, Roger with his addiction undertook to recover from a face-lift. Therefore all my advance concern for how long I would have to stay out of the sun. Therefore all the cheating when I was still black-and-blue. The early morning brief toastings seated on the benches in front of Louis and on Commonwealth Avenue, the quick lunch outdoors at Louis' cafe, the once-or-twice spread-eagled on the porch of the Braithwaites' house, the short runs to the airport with the sunroof open. In my heart I knew I had overdone it, knew I must suffer, knew sunbathing had caused the raccoon rings.

Yet—there was one missing piece. And now it would be supplied. Since Dr. Kaswell would not admit to seeing any problem, let alone explain it, I sought out an expert in whom I had the greatest confidence: Basil Sell.

Dermatologists, like cosmetic surgeons, train themselves to notice nothing out of the way when a patient first comes in, lest they make the patient aware of some horror that had escaped notice. You could go in with a maxillary tumor the size of a cucumber and they would say: "What is it that bothers you?" But Sell is a truth-teller, and when I told him what bothered me, Sell did not pretend to be unable to see it.

He asked for the list of my medications and, when he heard Minocin, said: "Minocin, if taken over a long time, can darken the skin. How long have you been taking it and how much?"

"Three years, ten milligrams a day."

"That's a lot. Who prescribed it and what for?"

I thought Sell himself had prescribed it at a time when I was troubled by a little outbreak of adult acne. However, a check of the records showed not. Once, when Sell had been too busy for an immediate appointment, I had seen a younger associate, and it was this associate who had prescribed the Minocin—with unlimited refills.

"But have you been having any acne?"

"No, but I always think I might have—especially if I have an important lecture to give and feel under stress because of it."

"You've been taking a drug for three years because you worried about getting a pimple you never got?"

I hung my head.

Dr. Sell looked at the discoloration with magnifying glasses. "These are *not* bruises. If they were they would be some shade of chartreuse by now. This is black pigment, and it is caused by Minocin."

"But why does it follow the raccoon-mask pattern, which I didn't have before the face-lift?"

"I don't know for sure, since I've never seen this kind of thing or heard of it, but I have a theory. The Minocin somehow interacted with the operation, and discoloration occurred only where both were active. Hence the pattern of the mask."

"What about the sun?"

"People on Minocin should be careful about the sun but the risk of a burn is much less than with tetracycline. Still, it's not zero. With your heavy tan and protective pigmentation, you had no trouble with Minocin alone. But then, add the trauma of a face-lift, and you get pigment just in the area all three factors operate: Minocin plus sun plus trauma."

"I guessed," I told Sell. "I stopped taking Minocin a week ago." I might have said with Hamlet: "O my prophetic soul!" I had known all along but thought I could escape the consequences.

"It's a good thing, and you mustn't take any more of it. But, cheer up! The darkening produced by Minocin goes away. It takes months, though. You should look better by the time school starts. By Christmas it will be almost gone. Eventually it should all go away."

I almost kissed his hands. "Thank you for inventing so merciful a theory—a theory with hope in it."

Sell smiled. "I even believe it."

And Sell's predictions came to pass. By September I looked better. I could still clearly see the discoloration, but even Jack wasn't able to.

And no one ever told me I looked rested. But returning students said something better: "Have you seen Professor Brown? He looks wonderful." And that made me feel something good might still be in store for me.

Chapter 5

Skippy

"You are a very nice man. Thank you for a great time, Skippy." I found the note propped against the telephone on Friday after Edwige had been in to clean. For a few seconds, I could not imagine what it meant or where it had come from. "You *look* like a Skippy," I had said to the boy I saw Sunday afternoon, August 17, 1991.

"That's cool; that's what my friends call me." He was wearing a blue baseball cap and a red satin B.U. baseball jacket much too large for him but draped in a way that looked sort of fashionable, yet boyish. Skip was twenty-four years old but looked eighteen. He must have put that small, warm note somewhere for me to find it, but it remained hidden until Edwige turned it up.

I missed the note but had not failed to think of Skip. Our time together had not been so great–and yet it had been. Skip leaned his head back, closed his eyes, and accepted endless deep kisses, beatific as a nursing babe, and that was wonderful, but he became erect only very briefly.

"I loved seeing you, but I'm disappointed in myself that I didn't arouse you."

"Are you kidding? Fresh flowers, beautiful paintings, and you sucked my dick. What's not to like? I had a great time."

With both hands, in the polite Japanese manner, I handed him an envelope: "That's three hundred dollars," eighty dollars over the agency fee.

And then, for the first time, Skippy turned on me his concerned, puzzled look and the direct blue-eyed gaze that went with it. "That's a lot. Are you sure?" And behind him he left the memory of that look and the note–like a fortune in a fortune cookie.

The second time Skip appeared at my door he brought from behind his back a small bouquet of red roses and baby's breath. I recognized the flowers from an outdoor stand that stood next to the subway exit. "Thank you. That's very sweet of you."

Later on, naked in bed, Skip lay on his stomach, his butt slightly elevated, and poked his penis down between his legs, like a second bouquet, so that I might see that it was slightly hard and surprisingly large. I took off the boy's white socks, one at a time, and sucked his toes, really sucked them, running my tongue between them, all the while stretching out one arm to finger his butt, dipping in and out a short distance. Nobody had an orgasm that day, but everybody had a good time.

The first two visits from Skip were in the same period as the last two from another d.b. In a cynical smart-ass mood I would say that I liked to have a second boy in the bullpen, warming up, but there was really no such calculation in it; it just happened that way.

For Skip's predecessor, I had bought in The Sharper Image a leather athletic bag with a large number of zippered compartments, costing just under $100, and that had been the gift he liked the best—by far. It was pronounced "really cool." For Skip's third visit I bought another such bag.

"Holy shit! I can't believe you bought this for me." Skip was one of the few people in the world who could convince you that he was truly thrilled with your gift. A few days later came a note: "I used my gym bag today. It has room for all of my shit. And I have really got shit!! I would never have bought anything so beautiful for myself."

It was on the third visit also that I said: "It's clear that you don't feel comfortable with me sexually, never have really. I'm not going to worry about that. I value you for yourself; sex isn't important, though I wouldn't want us to give up all physical intimacies. I don't want to lose you over erections or orgasms."

"That's very generous," and Skip looked shy and appreciative.

And so it became clear that my problem was emotional loneliness and that the cure for this, though linked to sex, was separable from it. Emotional loneliness is also separable from social loneliness. After Al's death our friends had rallied round with plenty of invitations; I need never have eaten my dinner alone or spent a solitary evening. But company, I found, was almost irrelevant. It was not entirely so. It

is worse to be emotionally lonely with no place to go than emotionally lonely with lots of people seeking your company.

My loneliness, though it was greatly intensified by Al's death,
preceded the death by some years; years in which Al too had been
lonely. In the months when Albert was dying I was usually with
him, every evening and weekend going to the doctor or to the
emergency room, but, in a deeper sense, Al died alone. And that
was probably the reason why the photographs taken on our tour of
the Far East caught an expression of terror on Al's face. He was
alone in his final Passion because the two of us had lost the ability
to get through to one another in a deep way.

For this I blamed Albert more than myself, because he told me
that all the men in his family were the same; they lacked the ability
to be tender and the wives complained about it.

Had it always been that way, even when we were young? It was
hard to be sure, because we were so often united in sexual passion.
But in the intervals between, something was lacking. After making
love Albert would turn his back, and I would lie against him and
hold him, but I could not with certainty remember being caressed. I
could, with certainty, remember thinking myself in some ineradica-
ble way unlovable. And when I remembered these things they were
hard to forgive, and they made it easier to get over the death.

There was one tiny strange exception. Something never discussed, something that might not have been an intended communication at all but just random movement. After the two of us had
made love and were lying together, Al's fingers, in contact with my
skin, would sometimes twitch slightly in an unpatterned way, as if
to convey a heavily coded message from deep within. And I, inten-
tionally, would twitch back, doing my best to duplicate the style as
if to say: "I read you. I don't know why your message must be so
covert and scrambled, but I have it and I take it for a sign of love."

Not everyone who was willing, and not very many who were
interested, could assuage my loneliness. Women were the most willing but none could help. It seemed that only handsome young men
were qualified and only a very few of them. A large number looked
as though they could help, but then they would say or do something
that made them as useless as women. So it had really been necessary

for me to screen a large number of good-looking young men, a large number of possibly qualified nonapplicants, a roster of dream boys.

My susceptibility—or should I say vulnerability—to expressed tenderness had been the cause of my one serious affair in Al's lifetime. I was forty and the boy, whose name was Rick, was twenty. Rick was, and the term was his, a "hair-burner." He was also blond and very beautiful. I could still summon the image caught in a mirror of a bedroom in New York City of Rick paddling in an oversize bathtub, an unself-conscious, adorable white pollywog. After the first three weeks Rick said: "Are you getting serious? Because I'm falling in love."

He had a gift for expressing feeling. When I was driving at night, for instance, Rick would lie on his back in the front seat, his head in my lap. When we went to the movies he held my hand. Simple stuff, but new and wonderful to me.

After nine months Rick and I parted without anger, mostly over differences connected with age. Al had put up with the whole thing, never jealous, he insisted, but often angry at my lack of consideration. When it ended Al said: "Why don't we try again?" And of course I wanted to. But for a long time afterwards I wondered how I could live without what Rick had given me.

Skippy did not just alleviate my loneliness, he eliminated it, and my heart sang as it had not since the early months with Rick. I myself never asked why I should have fallen in love with Skippy, never asked why Skippy should be the one, only the third in my lifetime, to arouse that almost psychotic happy obsession we call "falling in love." It was because Skippy was special. The whole cause lay in the object. My friends could not quite see the specialness. Gregg, looking at a picture, said: "Very pretty." Jack disliked Skip at the start. Edwige said: "He's fun." Rebecca, for whom all true love must be eternal, said: "He's like a young Al."

For Dodie in Berlin and Cheryl in Baltimore and Barry in New York City, who could not see Skip, I tried to describe his charms. Skip and I had been to a revival of *Bye Bye Birdie*, which we liked a lot, and when the audience applauded, Skip jumped up on his seat and whistled—an ear-splitting, two-fingers-in-the-mouth whistle. I tried conceptualizing the charm in this. "It's not easy for me to feel such enthusiasm and excitement, but I can participate in his."

Skip would sometimes interject in conversation: "Does anyone mind if I fart?" or would jump up and run out saying: "I have to pee" or "I have to go poopee." When we stayed together at the Pierre in New York he might say: "I have to take an enormous dump" and afterwards: "It was the size and shape of Uganda." Where's the charm? My conceptualization: "Everything about his body is ego-syntonic. He loves everything about his body, and this, combined with his freshness and beauty, is captivating." I once asked Skip why he talked so much about his "natural functions"– that distanced phrase is mine and goes a long way toward explaining Skip's appeal in this domain.

In the streets, whenever a dog came along, Skip would drop into a crouch and romp and pet and nuzzle and call the dog "puddin'." It was the same with the horses in Central Park; they also were petted and fawned over and called "puddin'." The only human Skip ever called "puddin' " was me. Not at first. At first he asked: "What shall I call you?" and rejected both "Doc" and "Rog" in favor of "Roger." After three months or so, when we walked anywhere, Skip, always in the lead, would pull on an invisible leash and call back to the professor: "Come on, puddin'! Come on." With an intonation suited to a Pekinese.

In *Les Miserables* there was something that reminded him of his childhood and he cried all through the show. I tried to make contact with this intense inner life, but Skip shook me off. I had not earned the right to touch the deep place from which it came. After the show, walking crosstown back to the Pierre, Skip strutted down the middle of the street singing the songs as loud as he could. Passersby loved it and so did I.

With every waiter, salesperson, and elevator operator Skip immediately created a personal relationship–usually with a compliment. He once told me that he had been good at his job as a callboy because he could always read the fantasy in a client's face–whether it was marriage and a white picket fence or advanced S & M. He seemed to be able to do that with everyone, and he was so generous as to feed the fantasy in even the briefest encounter. There is a young man operating an elevator in the Hotel Pierre who probably counts among the highlights of his life his four encounters with Skip. Skip unerringly identified this man's best feature–very white teeth and a good smile–and praised it so extravagantly that, as I cautioned Skip, he probably expects to ride to fame and fortune on his smile alone.

Skippy's "field," as one might say, was intimate relationships. Not studying them or conceptualizing or theorizing about them, but having them, creating them, and transforming them. Nothing else interested him very much. He would say: "I'm not a very political person," but very few who heard it can have guessed it meant he did not read a daily newspaper or watch the news on television. He had little interest in what was going on in the world. Once, at my apartment on a Sunday morning with a few minutes to kill, he picked up the newspaper and chose to look at the comics.

About a month after meeting me, Skippy got a regular job as a legal aide in the office of a man who had once been in love with him, and he quit the callboy agency. He never spoke of his work at all; he seemed to do it well enough but it did not interest him. He did speak of the people at the office and of his relationships with them. Skippy did not conceive of himself as having a career and, when pressed by me about the future, said: "I had an old dream about going to law school." But this had no reality. He had honor grades from a little-known college, and he did very little reading.

His passion, he would say, was music. His beloved grandfather had paid for piano lessons, and Skip composed songs, both words and music. He also sang in a high sweet tenor. Not able to write music, he preserved the songs by taping them. He had no clear plans for "doing something" with his music and seemed to be content that occasionally, in a bar, a stranger would weep over one–a stranger who, more than likely, was using this means to get into Skippy's pants.

The music that was Skippy's passion was based on intimate relationships. Each song, and all of his songs were sad, was inspired by a former lover. He called himself the Terminator. Skippy said he'd made something lasting of each lover by turning him into music. I used to think it sounded as if each one, starting at the feet, became a pillar of saccharin.

My friends who heard all these things about Skippy said they could understand my infatuation. "He does not treat you with any deference, and that pulls him out of the student mold. He has none of the middle-class qualities you know in yourself and your friends. He is beautiful, pitiable, spontaneous, and romantic. He is really an exotic for you."

It did not occur to me until very late in the game to ask Skip: "Why did I fall in love with you?" The answer I got was the best that occurred to anyone: "Probably because of the way I can show feeling."

What Al could not do, what many cannot do, Skip could do surpassingly well. I once said to Rebecca: "What that boy doesn't know about making love is not worth knowing." And this was without serious genital involvement because we never tried that again. I once said: "My God, Skip, how wonderful you must be when you are in love, when you are this wonderful not in love."

What did Skip and I do together on the many evenings in my apartment? You might say we played sex games, or we engaged in prolonged imaginative foreplay that never proceeded to consummation, or that we just "hung out" in an intimate way. Sometimes Skip would call out: "Time to get naked!" And he would, naked as a jaybird, though my sense of the age difference kept me from doing the same. Skip would turn the lights out and run a tub and get in and I would come in with a single lighted candle. There would be talk and jokes and I might stroke the boy's butt or reach for his genitals, and Skip would dodge away, though the intent was understood not to be serious.

Long after the sex games were over an abstract formulation occurred to me. They had been like scenes of father-son sexual molestation, rendered safe. Whether Skip and his father had such games I never knew. I played the father, pressing for sex, and Skip was the son, teasing, but drawing back. But with us it was only play, because both knew that the last thing we wanted was actual consummation.

The best part of the bathtub game was staring deeply into one another's eyes. I would rest my chin on the edge of the tub and Skip would turn on his side to face me and we would stare. It was unlike any ordinary eye contact. Neither felt any uneasiness or need to look away. We seemed to plumb one another's souls. It was the gaze of the lover, though we were not lovers. Even in our worst times later on I could not believe that it meant nothing, that Skip was only turning in a performance. After a long gaze I might say: "You'll miss me when I'm gone," and Skip would frown and say: "Why should you ever be gone?"

"Do you really not know that I am bound to be gone before long?"

Sometimes we spread a quilt on the living-room floor and lay down to watch a movie together. Skip would rest his head on my chest and take one of my hands. For me the action was not in the movie; in fact, I would lose track of the story and have to ask Skip, who always knew. The drama that mattered to me lay in Skip's nonverbal signals. They were never perfunctory, as they are in less gifted communicators. There would be squeezings and shifts of position and transfer of hands and intervals of gazing in profoundly meaningful patterns which resist verbal paraphrase.

The apogee of movie bliss came on Halloween ("Halloweenie" to Skip). The master communicator surpassed himself, but something happened that disturbed me, only a little at the time but a lot later on. Between films (*Popcorn* and *Dracula*) Skip jumped up, saying: "I better call Jim." Jim was a chief petty officer in the Navy, about thirty-five years old, who had befriended Skip when he first came to Boston two years earlier, and in ways never specified, helped him when he was without resources. Skip called on the bedroom phone and I overheard only one loud angry outburst: "Where am I? I'm out!" As he coolly nestled back into place beside me he said: "Jim's such a weenie."

I knew that Jim and Skip were not lovers, not at present anyway. Later on Skip let slip the information that he sometimes slept over at Jim's, in the same bed and naked. He sometimes did the same with his pal Groovy. My nerves had never permitted me to sleep with anyone, so this sounded almost more intimate than sex. Skip attempted to reassure me by saying: "Of course we don't make love; we just hold hands and stuff like that."

What a pity it is that people must always come with a history and with prior attachments. Or, given that they always must, what a pity that we do not enjoy them when they are with us and be otherwise incurious. But we cannot and, if anyone could, it would not be dear, possessive, and jealous Roger.

Skip came with as little history as a twenty-four-year-old can have. He had adored his mother, who had been an alcoholic and had died of drink. Once, in the early weeks, after some gifts that hit the "Holy shit!" level on Skip's Richter scale, he asked me: "Who sent you? My mother sent you, didn't she?"

Skip's father was then in his late fifties, almost twenty years older than Skip's mother. He was a handsome man and a smooth talker who had always charmed the ladies. In fact, however, he despised women and their sexuality. He had tortured his wife with paranoid accusations of infidelity and admired Skip's manly, robust sexuality. When it became clear that the sexuality was directed toward men, the father's anger drove the son from home.

Skip once said of his music that what he most hoped for was that a song of his might reach some unhappy kid and give him hope. This unhappy kid would be gay, filled with self-doubt and guilt, oppressed by his family, and, not perhaps essentially, but at least incidentally, reasonably cute. Very probably Skip's sympathy for puppy dogs and horses and any person in a serving capacity was part of the same complex. As were all his little-boy things: a "rubber duckie" (his phrase) for the bathtub game, Mickey Mouse Band-Aids, stuffed animals. Perhaps also the confidence that his pee and his poopee could give no offense. The entire setup derived from his own sad time as a powerless boy. In any case, it was clear that older and more powerful persons were excluded from the set that enjoyed his sympathy. "I don't feel sorry for you, Roger," he said, at a time when some would have.

Another time, Skip said: "I am like a moth or firefly always sending out the signal: 'You can fuck me but you have to love me too.'" The relevance of that striking remark to Skip's relation to other young men was clear to me, as also was my own profound, ultimate irrelevance to the boy who said it.

In addition to Skip's mother and father there were a stepmother and a brother. Skip said he loved them but, to an outsider, they did not seem to be very important. Probably Skip had many friends, but just two seemed to matter. There was Jim, his best friend, of whom Skip once said: "I think he'd like to flush me out of his system but I guess he can't." And there was Groovy, Skippy's own age, with whom he hung out and smoked pot and went to movies. Groovy was, in his own words, "always there for him." To me it seemed that Groovy, like Jim, was helplessly in love with Skip, and in a sexual way at that.

Why should a boy who, on casual contact, charmed just about everyone have just two friends, and those two bound by an unreciprocated physical attraction? Impossible to know, but the answer had something to do with Skip's sexuality. In one of his bathtub confidences he told me that he usually masturbated five times a day. At the gym, where he worked out every day, he often picked up or was picked up by someone to have sex. In his two trips to New York with me, Skip was snapped up on his first night almost as soon as the sun went down. Barry, my young friend in New York with a lot of experience, pronounced Skip "sexuality incarnate." In conversation, with people of all kinds, Skip dominated whenever he could turn the topic to sex, and he usually could. When he could not, as at George and Steve's Christmas bash, he just dropped out. He always noticed physical beauty in males or females and commented on it. Whether a man had a large penis was the most important thing to know about him.

All of the above are true of many young gay men, but the rest is not. Skip never took part in threesomes or steamroom orgies; it was always one-on-one. Skip never had anything to do with bathroom sex or glory holes. Sex was making love for him, one whole person with another whole person. His *frequent* sex was not *casual* sex. It was part of a quest, an unremitting quest for the right person who would fuck him well and also love him well. When someone proved unsatisfactory in either respect, and partner after partner did, Skip cut him off. He would not settle for anything less than complete fidelity. Otherwise, Termination! It was also himself he cut off, because Skip's "ex'es," and there were many of them, stayed in love with him and eventually found it too painful simply to be friends.

I once suggested to Skip that his quest for a lover was too relentless—that he ought to go about other kinds of business, as most people do, and let it happen when it would. "Love is an obsession with you."

"But it's the most important thing in life, isn't it?" Skip had me there.

How did Skip come to have any friends at all? There were just those who loved him too much, those willing to give up any sexual claims and selflessly adore him. There were only the two, Jim and Groovy, but Skip could do with more and I seemed to be qualified.

I was not qualified to be a lover. I myself knew this best. I barely made it as a make-believe lover and, indeed, did not make it without some scene setting and stage management. The first time we had dinner together–Skip brought over his homemade meatloaf–Skip asked me if I had any candles, which I did not, and he unscrewed a couple of lightbulbs in the kitchen fixtures. Was creation of romantic ambiance the point? I came to think it was to find that low level of illumination at which the defects of age and disfigurement should be faint enough to enable Skip to sustain the magical lover's gaze.

I took to buying candles in colors that complemented the fresh flowers on the coffee table and lighting the living room with just candles and one dim lamp. For our bathtub trysts, Skip instructed me to turn out the harsh overhead lights and come in with a single candle. One evening the lighting arrangements struck me as so comical that I snuffed out my candle and said: "I don't look bad in the pitch dark."

For several months in the fall Skip and I always met at my apartment around seven, when the sun would be down. We did not meet in daylight until the morning of the first trip to New York in October. Skip had arrived ahead of time: "I'm too excited to wait! I hardly slept at all!" On the plane he stared out the window, listened to his music on the earphones, and looked a little downcast. I was feeling dashing in sunglasses with my tan in good shape, and asked if anything was wrong. Skip, frowning a bit: "It's just that we look so *different*." And of course, we did; Roger at sixty-six and Ivy League; Skip at twenty-four, something like Little League. Probably Skip had seen the reflection in the mirror, but while I had seen a distinguished diplomat in attendance on a young prince, Skip had seen–what? Something shockingly at variance with the illusion of our after-dark intimacy.

"Roger, do you have a neurological disorder?"

"What! No, of course not. What are you talking about?"

"Well, there's blood coming out of your ear."

I had cut myself shaving.

Eventually we got used to one another. In an optical store on Lexington Avenue, where we went so that Skip could buy several pairs of glasses–for cosmetic purposes–Skip bounced around charming all the salespeople. One woman asked him: "Who's that man with you?" and Skip answered: "That's my grandfather. He's ninety years old! Isn't he wonderful for his age?" This was so outrageous that I laughed and told the story many times.

On our second New York trip in our suite at the Pierre, I had elegantly entertained half a dozen people with catered canapes and champagne and Skip had taken it in. Two nights later I went to see Corigliano's opera *The Ghosts of Versailles* at the Met and Skip asked whether he might entertain, in the manner he had seen, two girls from his high school graduating class. I did not get in until 11:30, but to my dismay the three were still there, sipping champagne, and so introductions had to be made. With a flourish Skip said "This is Dr. Roger Brown, my travelling psychiatrist. He goes with me everywhere," and the girls could not think of a question. I could not think at all.

Skip and I went to see *Something for the Boys*, sitting in the third row, which Skip favored as he liked to put his feet up on the seat ahead and feel the movie wash over him. I gamely tried to do the same but my very long legs and my very big feet made it difficult. "Uh-oh," Skip said, straightening up and bringing his feet to the floor. Just behind him sat two of Skip's acquaintances, age-mates, and so boys. I sat upright in my winter overcoat, feeling like Daddy Warbucks caught molesting Little Orphan Annie. Skip introduced me but could not hit on anything better than, "This is Dr. Roger Brown." I supposed the "Dr." vaguely suggested a connection that was medical rather than sexual.

Why did Skip bother with the old professor? There was, of course, a financial aspect; with Skip no longer working as a callboy, I suggested: "Why don't we stabilize our financial relationship? I'd like to put you on a retainer of $500 a week."

"Why do you feel you have to give me money?"

"I don't feel I have to. I love you and I want to make your life easier. You give me a chance to be generous. I admit that I would buy you if I could, but you aren't for sale."

The checks were always in envelopes with cards and Skip would say: "Oh, you wrote something for me! What's this, more dollars? I don't know what to do with it all." In fact the retainer, which Skip called his "salary," was almost exactly the small salary he was paid on his job and almost half what I made.

The cards I wrote were sincere: "You are the sunshine of my life. What can repay sunshine?" "On days when I am going to see you my heart sings."

On November 7, however, I copied out the whole of Sonnet No. 29:

> When in disgrace with fortune and men's eyes
> I all alone beweep my outcast state
> And trouble deaf heav'n with my bootless cries,
> And look upon myself and curse my fate.
> Etc, etc.
> Haply I think on thee, and then my state,
> Like to the lark at break of day arising
> From sullen earth, sings hymns at heaven's gate;
> For thy sweet love remembered such wealth brings,
> That then I scorn to change my state with kings.

In response Skip wrote: "Thanks for the card and $—I must admit I'm about as much in touch with Shakespeare as I am with my scrotum."

The cryptic reference to being in touch with his scrotum is a reference to the first New York trip, the trip of late October, and that event must now be related and, in chronological order, five others which led to the final crisis.

* * *

The idea for a sumptuous weekend à deux in New York began with my interest in seeing Puccini's *Girl of the Golden West*, an opera I had never seen and which was being given by the Met in the fall of 1991. In mid-October I asked Skip whether he would be interested. Would he! Skip's eyes shone. He had loved the bits of *La Bohème* played in the movie *Moonstruck,* and an older gentleman of earlier acquaintance had promised Skip some day to take him to see *La Bohème* but had defaulted on this promise. Months later I heard more about the older gentleman—a smarmy, defrocked priest—stuck on *La Bohème.*

"Well, *Girl of the Golden West* is by the same composer as *Bohème:* Puccini. It's much less melodious and less popular than *Bohème,* but you might like it."

"I want to go! I want to go! It would be a dream come true. I lived in New York for a few months and I loved it. Please, Roger, can we go?"

"I think it would be fun to stay at the Pierre, which I liked a lot last spring. We could take a suite with two bedrooms and baths and so each have our privacy. You can wear your dark suit, Skip, and you'll be the best-looking man in that glamorous audience."

Tickets for the opera, the premiere of a new production, were sold out but Barry and Anthony, who live in New York, told me that there was a way to get tickets to anything: an illegal scalping agency. I called and found I could get two good seats for $500 each. They could also get tickets to *Les Miserables.*

"Would you want to stay an extra day and see *Les Miserables?*"

"I would give my left nut to see *Les Miserables!* Roger, you are amazing! And a prince!"

At the opera Skip sat next to a great Opera Dragon, eighty years old, hair piled a foot high, hands encrusted with jewels.

"Are those real?" Skip asked. The Dragon took a good long look at the boy and his escort and hit on the correct answer instantly. I made upper-class opera discourse with her and Skip whispered to me: "The old broad is playing footsie with me."

My hopes for the opera had been that Skip and I would experience synchronous musical thrills, breathing sighs with tear-filled eyes, and be drawn together in a new way. The first opportunity *Girl of the Golden West* provides for a big thrill is the Wild West motif that booms from the orchestra with Minnie's entrance into the Polka Dot Saloon. I sought to cue Skip by taking a breath so deep that the boy should feel the chest expansion. But Skip was otherwise engaged—gnawing his nails to the cuticle. The opera was killing him, and later on he swore he would never go again.

At the first intermission we spotted a group of gay men, including Christopher, a boy of Skip's age whose lambent gaze fixed on us and never moved. Skip thought he was being "hit on."

"Why should you assume that he's looking at you? It's me he's interested in."

"You're so funny," Skip said.

At the second intermission Skip and I had a drink with the gay men who, excepting Christopher, were all hard-looking New York queens in their forties and fifties. Christopher was being kept by the ugliest one who was, incidentally, HIV positive.

"I don't suck his dick or anything," Christopher whispered to Skip.

"I can't have sex with you," Skip whispered back. "Roger might commit suicide if he knew."

Leaving the opera house, one of the New York men hissed at me: "Good night, sugar daddy."

Now that the opera ordeal was over, Skip came vividly to life and knew exactly what he wanted—to take a taxi to a Village bar called Uncle Charlie's, where he had often gone with Kendall—"the only man I ever loved." Skip had these histrionic, silent-movie name tags for the significant people in his life ("Jim, my best friend" "Groovy, a saint"), and he repeated them on every conversational entry, as inevitably as Homer's *Epithets.*

I had heard quite a lot about Kendall before—but nothing about Skip's private agenda for this trip, which was to exorcise Kendall's ghost by revisiting all the major sites and saying good-bye.

The taxi driver found the Village but not Uncle Charlie's. He repeatedly opened his window to the rainy night and inquired the way. Because the driver was Chinese and because New Yorkers require brevity, the inquiry came out: "Uncle Cholly?" with a high-rising intonation. It was seldom understood and endlessly repeated, and Skip took it up as a routine, good for a laugh anytime at all as long as the trip lasted. Afterward it became part of the shared culture of Skip and myself.

"What part of your body are you least in touch with?" was the beginning of another routine that entered our culture. The answer was "my scrotum." Skip created this one also and, as we have seen, found it useful for describing his remove from Shakespeare.

Like Skip, I was clear about what I wanted to do after the opera—go straight to bed. However, I was a good sport until we had been at Uncle Charlie's for an hour and it was 1:30 a.m., quite late enough to trigger my sleep panic. Skip was deep in conversation with some swarthy, unsuccessful musician who was giving the impression that he could advance Skip's musical career—to what end, we already know.

"I'm tired and I'm going back to the hotel."

Skip followed me out to look for a cab and Skip's hot-eyed suitor followed him. As I stepped into a cab: "Are you sure?" And there it was—the concerned slight frown and clear blue gaze that I knew. Of course it never occurred to Skip to go back with me. It was only 1:30 and this was New York!

Next morning I at last blew up. Skip was on the phone talking to last night's bedmate and had been for almost an hour.

"I can't believe it! You dumped me last night, our first in New York, and now you're doing it again! Ordinary decency should tell you better! Get out! Get out of my room!" And I waved an arm.

Skip immediately darted out. Long afterwards I remembered the instant response to my raised arm, which must have seemed to threaten violence. I remembered it later when Skip told me his father used to abuse his mother. I remembered it later when I learned that Skip's 210-pound lover, Vin, was abusive.

But I never hit anyone. Instead I analyzed and talked and eventually decided the fault was mine: "Because I just cannot remember how old I am."

"How old *are* you?" the boy asked, as if expecting the answer to be obscene.

And my anger was turned into another comedy routine by Skip and added to the common culture under the name "flying into a rage!" And Skip would perform it, rolling his eyes and gnashing his teeth.

The last night Skip got in around four and drew a bath and for about an hour happily sozzled in the oversize bathtub ("as big as the Grand Canyon") in the overpriced suite in the luxury hotel and thought how he might never see its like again.

When I got up much later I found in the hall of the sitting room two cheap, flamboyant neckties and this note:

Good morning!
Bought us matching ties. Thanks for the
awesome weekend.
I said goodbyes—
I said hellos
I had a fucking blast!
Skippy

Back in Boston in the cab, Skip kept his distance and looked sullen, not just tired, but sullen. I could not, at first, figure out what was the matter. And then it came to me that Skip still thought as a callboy thinks, that he thought of the New York weekend as Gennaro had thought about the projected-but-not-realized Provincetown weekend. He had given up three working days and so lost income for which he should be compensated. I took $400 from my wallet—nearly emptying it—and forced it into Skippy's hand. Skip then scribbled a note.

> You are very special to me. This weekend was a very memorable experience—I want you to know that my feelings go beyond $—please remember that. You are a true friend. *First* and foremost.

> Skippy

* * *

The first of my friends to whom I introduced Skip were Sue and Peg, a lesbian couple. I chose them because they were smart, good-looking, youngish (in their forties), lively, and, in every way, *cool*. Also because they loved and admired me and would be sure to tell Skippy he was lucky to have snared such a paragon. Lesbians, we know, simply do not understand the ageism of gay men, which decrees that no virtues whatever can make sixty-six-year-old Roger a suitable lover, though perhaps a "good catch" for twenty-four-year-old Skip.

Immediately upon being introduced, Skip took Sue's face in his hands and then Peg's and said: "You're so beautiful. Are you really lesbians?"

Peg was an openly gay member of the Cambridge City Council and very well acquainted with all the Cambridge neighborhoods. After dinner she led the way to the Kendall Square Bar, a modest corner bar with entertainment. Skip was struck with the name "Kendall," corresponding as it did with that of "the only man I ever loved," and took the omen to be good.

It was a very quiet night in the Kendall Square Bar—about ten paying customers—and members of the audience were encouraged

to come to the microphone and sing a number. Peg and Sue and I
started clapping and calling Skip's name and a good-natured couple
nearby joined in. Eventually he complied.

The boy's professional manner was a little surprising even to one
who knew him so well. (It was at once more self-assured than
expected and less confident.) The self-assurance was a good imitation of a TV performer but there was a shakiness, not entirely
concealed, that seemed to say he was ready to bolt if anyone was
unfriendly. No one was, and he got a good hand and did an encore.
The large jolly woman in charge of the bar, a Sophie Tucker type,
complimented Skip on his talent and invited him to do a full set
some evening. The date fixed on was December 12. It was understood that the debut was an "opportunity" and so, naturally, would
be unremunerated.

I worried about the debut. Not about Skip's ability to carry it off
but about what kind of figure I myself might present. Skip was
inviting all his friends and I pictured something like a Who concert:
young, exuberant, noisy. And, in their midst, myself. An elderly man
with the wrong clothes and the wrong expression on his face. Probably they would call me names and pelt me with breadsticks.

Above all, Skip and I must avoid any sign of having a "special
relationship," and so Skip would arrive early with "best friend"
Jim, and I would arrive near showtime with good-looking, straight-
looking Jack, who would put down Skip's crowd by virtue of his
masculine good looks.

Jack agreed to be the date, even though he had never liked Skip.
The idea was to prop me up in my vulnerable position. For Skip's
sake, and not just my own, I exacted definite commitments to attend
from everyone I felt I could ask: Edwige, Edwige's mother, Peg and
Sue, Rebecca, Gregg. And, since flowers and a good-luck card
would be opaque to the uninformed, I had two dozen white roses
delivered from Winston's.

On the evening of December 12, by the time I arrived, the full
invited audience could be assumed to be in attendance. On my side
of the aisle sat all the eight asked, on Skip's side were only Jim and
Groovy, and it was they, rather than Roger and company, who
appeared to feel awkward and out of place. I enjoyed a brief exulta-

tion, but this gave way to sympathy for brave Skip, who tossed off: "I guess my friends lost their invitations."

Skip never wrote a song *about* me as for all his former lovers; presumably I did not inspire that kind of music. Skip had, however, written a song *for* me in which he developed the poetic conceit that he was a mediator, a line of transmission from Albert. He closed his concert with this number.

Somewhere near
candles peel
light falls in on the unreal
and you are there
the night finds gold within your hair

where's the sound I need to hear
where's the song you want to sing
where's the man you hold so dear

somewhere near
every movement
every expression on your face was a word
silent passing
from here to here
but now, first it has to go through
me

for a moment he was me
for a moment he was me.

* * *

New York at Christmas almost makes up for New York the rest of the year; at least it does if you confine yourself to midtown Manhattan. There is a real feeling of excitement and generosity that brings people together. I imagined myself and Skip tooling along Fifth Avenue doing Gucci and Pucci. I imagined us in the hush of Christmas Eve walking in the snow, in our suite at the Pierre having breakfast together.

I was having almost weekly attacks of panic and they were all caused by the same thing: Skip's failure to phone. It had reached the point where I would grow tense a full two hours before the agreed-upon time, usually nine or thereabouts, close to my bedtime. The tension would grow and ten minutes before the hour I would feel sure the call was not going to be made, though I would not quite give up hope until an hour or two later. In the interval, many calls would come from persons other than Skip, and each "false positive" would create a cardiac leap of hope followed by an over-hasty conversation aimed at keeping the line open.

As the hour grew late, hectic attempts were made to reach Skip, in hopes of an explanation pacifying enough for the professor to compose himself for sleep. I might try Skip's beeper number; Skip always wore his beeper. A beeper displays the number calling and leaves the wearer the option of responding or not. I would imagine the boy languidly glancing at the display and choosing, in whatever bed or bordello, to let the old boy wait until morning. It was never possible to convict him of such heartlessness because he could just say, "My beeper must have been out." Beepers, one knew, often did not work.

If, instead of the beeper, I tried the home number, then I would get Sophie, Skip's landlady. She would solemnly promise to tell Skip to call when he came in, that very evening, however late. If no call came, either Skip had not come in at all or he had not bothered to call because Sophie was an alcoholic, always drunk in the evening. You could not count on Sophie. To me Skip seemed to be a master of telecommunications, like Klingsor in *Parsifal*, an evil magician in the center of a web he controlled.

In full-fledged panic and rage, I would at last turn out the lights, my mind racing until I knocked it out with sedatives and alcohol. Next day, feeling very rocky, I would end the relationship forever. But, given a plausible explanation, I would take it all back.

The very first time the cycle of panic, farewell, and forgiveness occurred was October, and I, after saying "good-bye forever," almost immediately began to regret it. By the time I left school at five I was thinking: "What is the matter with me? Am I hoping to find the Perfect Lover at age sixty-six? Now I've lost the only happiness in my life." When Skip eventually answered my repeated phone calls and forgave me I shakily said: "Thank God."

The first reconciliations were sweet and probably the tension and relaxation strengthened the bond. In November and December, however, the whole thing became almost routine, and painfully ignominious. It was all about missed phone calls, something utterly trivial and something that should easily be fixed. To me it seemed Skip just could not be bothered. To Skip it seemed I was an incredible pill. And to both our bond was looking drab. An exciting return to New York at Christmastime should help.

Skip found a card with an apt picture on it, a small boy "making a muscle" which a tall milkman was indulgently bending down to feel, and inside he wrote:

Roger
Skip
N.Y.C.
Again
God help the Pierre
Phantom
Saigon
Christmas
No Montana
Barry
Anthony
You
Are
Very
Special
To
Me

Phantom and *Saigon* were musicals we would see. "No Montana" was a reference to the fact, related to me after it was over, that Skip had had, for a short time, a suitor who wanted to carry him off to Montana, a proposal only recently declined. Barry and Anthony were young friends of mine, thirty-two and thirty-five respectively. Barry was a graduate student at Columbia, working on his PhD in the history of religion, and Anthony was a very junior member of a large law firm. Barry had been a protégé of Al's and, later on, a warm friend to both Al and me. When Al died I called Barry:

"We're creating our own funeral services. Cheryl and Rebecca will read poems and Dodie will read a beautiful piece she wrote for Al. Would you come and officiate, Barry?"

"You know I will."

Barry and Anthony had heard quite a lot about Skip, mostly about his charm. They were glad that he had drawn me out of mourning and back into life but concerned that he must eventually hurt me. They wanted to meet Skip and invited us to spend Christmas Eve, help decorate the tree, and share their supper. For me, the invitation was especially intimate and appealing, as it was for Skip, who picked up the special warmth on both sides.

Christmas Eve was our second evening in New York. Skip had had no sleep at all the first night because, once settled into the Pierre, there was nothing to do but fulfill my romantic wish to ramble the midtown streets, just the two of us, savoring the holiday spell, and this wish had no counterpart in Skip's mind. He was as restless and irritable as a cougar. I finally snapped: "Why don't you go out and get laid?"

"You mean it?"

"I can't stand spoiling your fun. I came here to be with you, and you came to have a blast."

"You knew how it'd be. What do you want?"

"I suggest you go out and get laid."

"You don't have to tell me twice."

Next morning Skip got in bed with me and, putting his arms around me, started to tell me what happened the night before. He met someone "incredibly beautiful, named John," and spent the night, and they both came three times. This much Skip got out before I could stop him.

"I can't believe you expect me to be your confidant in this." And I withdrew to the bathroom.

During the day Skip spent a lot of time in the ballroom of the Pierre, playing the grand piano. He was, he told me, composing a new song with the title "John Sleeping."

That evening with Barry and Anthony, to their immense embarrassment, Skip the Scamp told about meeting John, not omitting the fact that they had both come three times.

One must really ask what ailed me that I put up with it. Barry commented on the phone the next day: "Skip is sex incarnate, but you can see he has a real affection for you that's in some way sexual." We two had never been lovers in the full sense and I always took care to tell friends, "It would be indecent really." But as Skip once cheerily said: "We're not platonic either." There was plenty of ambiguity, yet anyone could see that what Skip was doing in New York was unconscionable. He saw it too. Perhaps he simply did not care enough to be deterred. And he knew he could always make up for it.

On Christmas Day Skip was morose. There seemed to be nothing to do in New York. Barry and Anthony had no more time for us. The suite at the Pierre looked pretentious and stupid.

Skip sighed and punched his pillow. The trouble was that John had not called. "I'm not going anywhere tonight. I'm just going to stay in and watch TV."

My foolish old heart jumped. Was Skip saying he wanted to spend the evening together? He wasn't. He turned off the lights and almost, but not quite, closed the door between our bedrooms, creating an impassable barrier behind which he sulked in silence.

After a mostly sleepless, very agitated night, I convinced myself that I was an irrelevancy in Skip's life, and decided that I could stand it no more. I wrote a note: "The bill is paid. I have to get out of this relationship, Skip. I wish I could stand it, but I can't." And I quietly packed my bags, intending to leave before Skip should awaken. But Skip was awake and ran to the old man and put his arms around him. "Don't leave, puddin'. I'm over John. We have all New York. Why leave? Let me unpack for you. We can have a beautiful day together."

And, incredibly, we did. We looked at the penguins in the Central Park Zoo, and Skip jumped around on the rocks singing at the top of his voice. We shopped for nothing in particular but bought a beautiful leather case for Skip in Le Vielle Russie, which caused him to say: "This is the second time today you've made me cry." A milky December sun shone and we petted all the dogs and all the horses. It was the kind of simple day that Skip could make magical.

The day ended with a snack at the Plaza, and we talked about what a strange pair we were, after all. Skip stood up, quite a small boy really in his too-large overcoat, and pointing dramatically at Roger, who was almost a foot taller but seated, said: "You belong to me."

* * *

"Are you doing anything New Year's Eve?"

"I guess I am now." But the implicit rebellion became explicit, and Skip told me he was spending New Year's Eve with his best friend, Jim, because he had not been seeing much of Jim lately. Skip did not immediately turn down an invitation to a New Year's Day brunch with Peg and Sue but he also did not commit himself.

"Are we going to brunch or not?"

"We're not."

This was the beginning of a period when Skip became mostly unavailable. The reasons given were various. The real reason was concealed. Skip had met Vin–a man his own age–and Skip and Vin were in love.

For Monday, June 6, Skip and I had a date to see the movie *Prince of Tides*, but Skip called to say that he felt sick–flu or something.

"Why don't I come out and see you for a few minutes?"

"Well . . . all right, I guess, if you really want to."

I had often dropped Skip off at the house in Dorchester but had never been inside. Dorchester is a tough Irish working-class neighborhood, not pretty to look at, but Macklin Avenue, where Skip lived, is different. The large old houses are set back on expansive lawns under broad shade trees, and on the outside the general effect is pleasant. Less so indoors, where borderline poverty shows in threadbare furnishings and lack of upkeep.

I arrived at seven with a modest nosegay of the kind Skip used to bring me. When I was introduced to Sophie–something I had not anticipated–I did a graceful conversion and presented the flowers to Madame. Sophie accepted with a coy smile and dropped into a half-curtsy, and I judged that I would stand high with her. Sophie's husband sat disconsolately drunk in the kitchen and did not look up on being introduced.

"This is my room," Skip said with some slight pride.

The first view of the room hit me like a punch in the stomach.

Dominating everything was an enormous TV, its metal cabinet painted black, its eye aimed at the punched pillows of a bed slung almost as low as a futon. On the bed, very rumpled, was a patch-work quilt of mine that Skip had admired and accepted as a gift with much joy. The TV picture was on all the time but not the sound. On the wall was a sample of Skip's artwork–two men's faces in generic comic-book style, faces totally empty of any life or expression. The shag rug was a gangrenous green, somewhat squishy underfoot, as if unimaginable small creatures lived there. In the entire room there was nothing to read.

"This is the bathroom. I share it with Danny. He's very good-looking and sweet but a little bit retarded. He's always after me to do something with him. Sometimes we take in a movie." There was no tub in the bathroom, which explained why Skip so loved to take a tub-bath at my apartment or, even better, at the Pierre, where he emptied into the water all the little tumblers of bath salts the hotel provides.

The poor kid, I thought. No wonder he has to get out of here every morning and stay away, using his beeper-and-telephone network to connect him with other people.

"These are my treasures; this is my dad."

"He's really handsome." He looked only about fifty years old.

"This is my mom."

"What a beautiful face."

"And this is my journal; I keep it locked. Look, here is your entry: 'Aug. 17. A really nice man; likes to kiss. I hope he calls again.' I gave you three stars. That's out of four."

After about ten minutes: "It was really nice of you to come. I appreciate it."

I had a strange feeling as I left that there was someone who could help Skippy with his flu but that it was not me. This was January 6; months later I learned that Skippy and Vin had first met on the fifth. I suggested we wait until January 8 to go to the movies, to give Skip a chance to get over his illness. Unfortunately, I called to make inquiries on the evening of January 7 and Skippy was out–all night as far as I could tell. I had one of my panics.

When Skip called on the eighth I felt too tired and humiliated to ask for an accounting.

"I know we planned to see *Prince of Tides*, but to tell the truth I don't really feel like it," Skip said.

"Then let's wait. I don't feel well myself. Let's not see one another until we both feel like it."

"What's wrong with you? You sound very low."

"The truth? I feel old and ugly and there isn't anything I can do about it. And I look particularly awful tonight."

From Skip there escaped a sound for which there is no transcription; almost a whimper, it expressed pained sympathy or pity.

"Why don't we go to the movie, puddin'? I can help you; I know I can. I don't care how you look."

The professor brightened a bit. "You missed a good chance. When I said I feel old and ugly, you should have said: 'You *feel* old and ugly? Honey, you *are* old and ugly.' "

Watching *Prince of Tides* from the third row Skip played on his companion a nonverbal accompaniment worthy of a Wurlitzer. The professor, all his defenses destroyed by fatigue, looked into the boy's eyes and said: "My God, how I love you."

"Me too." With a slight change of key: "In my fashion. Oh, you'll like the next scene; it's right where we were in the Central Park Zoo."

"How do you know? You've already seen the movie! It just opened so you must have seen it last night! That's where you were! Prince of Lies, that's you."

"Yeah, yeah, I've seen it but I was crazy about it and wanted to see it again."

"I'm sure you didn't see it alone. Jim, your best friend, as you always say, read the novel and predicted the movie would be the best movie this year."

Then, clearly telling the truth: "Roger, I didn't see the movie with Jim."

* * *

For the week of *Prince of Tides*, Skip suggested no additional appointments but said he would call on Sunday, January 12. I was not even surprised that that call, requiring memory over four days, was not made. Not surprised, but angry, and the failure stored as yet another grievance. Feeling bloodied and battered, I checked into the Ritz-Carlton for a few days.

Checking into the Ritz was something I did from time to time, very much as people sometimes sign themselves into McLean Hospital. The Ritz-Carlton had a soothing effect when one felt seriously ill-used. The name alone helped. The attractive and deferential, but not servile, staff made you feel liked and respected by some very nice people. And, of course, known by name.

I half-suspected that when I checked in, the good news swiftly went round among the staff: "The Professor is back." This should be so, because I was good at staying at the Ritz. I knew how to do it. I remembered names and made polite inquiries about families, and I looked the part. Very much the distinguished gentleman, each complimentary mirror and each smiling employee assured me.

I had formulated a few rules to maximize my own comfort and the comfort of the staff. For instance: "Do not do percentages to work out tips. Like a *grand seigneur,* tip as you list." I had once worked it out and found that careful attention to percentages, with all the attendant awkward delays, cognitive strain, and smudged erasures, resulted in a final saving of less than 5 percent. This being the case, I tipped ad lib. The intermittent positive reinforcement of occasional overtipping probably helped to account for my popularity with the hotel staff. And my *sprezziatura* undoubtedly won their admiration.

It is not surprising that I should have discovered the Ritz Hotel Self-Worth Fix, since the basic principle is the same as that of escort services. A human need, presently difficult to satisfy in usual ways, is satisfied, in purchasable ways. In Japan, one reads, it is possible to rent by the day an entire family, or any part of one, to satisfy unmet needs of kinship in an idealized way. Do you lack an indulgent grandmother or wish you had rebellious teenagers? There is an agency you can call. It may be the coming thing.

Skippy easily tracked me to the Ritz and, calling on the thirteenth, he suggested that we dine at the Ritz Cafe the next evening. When I was staying at the hotel, Skip would sometimes sharpen anticipation by leaving with the operator a message like "Skippy will be there at seven." On January 13 the message, delivered by an amused operator, was: "Put on your party pants. We're going out to dinner. Skippy." This being the most impudent message so far, it greatly charmed the professor.

Upon arrival at five, Skip told me that he would have to leave by 6:30 p.m. to get to a birthday party. This meant we would have to go into the dining room as soon as it opened at 5:30, when there would be no other diners there at all. It was a quiet dinner. I was furious and Skip's efforts to calm me failed. He tried to give the trembling old gentleman a taste of his snail soup. Not bloody likely. Skip promised to come again the following evening, for the full evening, but tonight he could not stay. No reply.

Back in my room at seven, I packed to leave and composed a message. Skip had recently added to his communications system a private line with a message machine. Vin, I would eventually learn, did not like going through either Sophie or the beeper. Skip had been reluctant to give the number to me but recently had done so.

"You filth, you scum!" I began. "I don't want to see you tomorrow or ever again." As it happened, the first line, so excellently expressive of my long controlled rage, was not recorded. The new machine somehow missed it and what it picked up was only the decisive but mild remainder. When I woke the following morning, after a very toxic night, I was horrified at having called Skip "filth" and "scum" because, while my words had often been implicitly threatening, I took some pride in never having been seriously abusive or wounding to a mere boy, a very vulnerable boy, a boy I loved. When I learned, as I did quite soon, that the disgraceful words had not been heard, I felt the greatest relief. I knew their impact, after all, because Albert had used them on me.

On Friday, January 17, a letter came. On the envelope there were none of the little stars and hearts that Skip customarily drew to express his blithesome nature and in the upper left corner not the usual absurd "Skippy" but a forbidding "R. W. Lowkie." And inside:

R,

Your telephone privileges are hereby suspended [highlighted in yellow]. If you ever again leave a message like the last one I will have the number changed [highlighted in red]. I don't

know what's going on inside your head but I don't want to see
you until you get over it.

The message was clearly intended to be very stern, but it struck
me as a child's conception of how to be stern. Still, I wondered at its
being as severe as it was, since "scum" and "filth" had not come
through and this was not, after all, the first time I had said "Good-
bye forever." Later on I would learn that in cancelling the Wednesday date I had caused Skip to miss out on an evening with Vin and
also to entangle himself in a net of lies that put strain on the new
romance, now already past its first bloom.

Skip's stern dismissal put me into a fever of composition.

Dear Skip,

You see I can still write "dear" even if you cannot. Your
ugly letter goes a long way toward making up my mind but it
does not quite do so because the stake after all is something
rare and valuable for both of us. So—
I don't think it is hard to get inside my head. I have turned it
inside out for you more than once. What I want is to be able to
love you more than anything else on earth. What is making
that impossible? Small things. You said you would call me last
Sunday but you did not. Trivial? It gave me a bad night and
started growing in me that old monster-jealousy. But I bit my
tongue and tried to ignore it.
Then on Tuesday, having encouraged me to expect a good
evening ("put on your party pants"), it comes out that we have
to go into the dining room as soon as it opens because you
must be off by 6:30 or so to a birthday party. So I feel dumped!
For the umpteenth time. You did offer limited sympathy: snail
soup from your own spoon and you would come again on
Wednesday. But then you had not previously spoken of coming over on Wednesday. So once again I feel like a john being
pacified. I am not a john, asshole! I love you—as much as
anyone ever will.
I understand that you will not curb your impulses, sexual or
social, for anyone and I sort of admire you for that. What I
cannot take is that you cannot be bothered even to do the

superficial things that would let me be at peace. If you say you will call, do it without fail. If you make a date with me, do not make a date that will cut me off early. Either don't make the date with me or tell me in advance what is up.

I am not asking for more intimacy, let alone sexual intimacy, nor that you give up your eternal quest for sex and/or romance. All I have ever asked is that you exercise a minimal consideration and forethought so that I can imagine that you care for me—with a high priority. Your insistence on self-determination is so great that you may not be able or willing to go along with such minimal rules. In which case I cannot stand it! I wish I could, but I am a sensitive and proud person and I cannot. It really can be managed, but I suspect you just cannot be bothered and, if so, I have to get out.

So, do you get it? I have endured a lot—being dumped at the Pierre, failure to make promised calls. And these things are hard on me—I am not young, as I think you may have noticed.

I am going into all this because I do not want to lose something I cherish because of misunderstanding. It has reached the point where, whatever the plan we make, I wait for the hitch to appear, the bomb to detonate. There is no happiness in this for me. Nor can I plan anything. I would like the two of us to go to some Caribbean island and tool around in a jeep. But maybe it's just not worth doing for you if you have to restrain your sexuality—even for a few days. On the other hand, as you saw at once, how would I control my jealousy?

I will tell it to you straight—my grand plan is to make you the center of my life. You have no grand plan; you enjoy each day and there is not much carryover from one to the next. Your life has a kind of beauty and I sort of admire it. Still I think you should control your impulses a bit, enough to keep me calm and in your life. Because it is a miracle that we found one another and what we have when the planets are all in orbit is wonderful. All it takes to make me relaxed and fun to be with is affection from you and no unhappy surprises or deception.

If this interests you, sweetheart, call me or write. If not, let it be.

Roger

Reading over my repetitious cry of the heart, I was disgusted. As Carmen says to Don José in Act IV: "A quoi bon tout cela. Entre nous, c'est fini." ("What's the use of all this? Between ourselves, it's finished.") The situation was clear and hopeless and different from that of Carmen and Don José only in that it had always been hopeless. I loved a pretty boy who could not, I knew, love me in return. What, then, was I asking? That the boy *endeavor* to love me? The futility of that is expressed in Bertram's line from *All's Well That Ends Well:* "I do not love the lady and cannot strive to do it." No one can strive to love; love is involuntary.

One really must wonder at Roger as he appears in this letter. He is pleading, not for love, but only for the pretense of love. No, not even for that much. But only for forbearance from actions that make it impossible to accept the semblance. How pusillanimous, how ignominious; what a wimp!

And yet, how full of grace Roger was in one respect. In everything he wrote or sent to Skip, the implication was that the boy ought to modify his behavior out of simple decency or compassion. And yet both Skip and he knew perfectly well that the main reason they were together at all was money. In never mentioning this, in never charging Skip with greed or ingratitude, Roger surely was magnanimous.

Or was he? Roger, as much as Skip, needed to believe that their relationship was more than the simple transaction: money for sex. If the relationship is seen as a transaction, Skip becomes a prostitute or whore and Roger becomes a john or a whoremonger. Unlovely terms for both and so both; have an interest in looking away from the financial aspect. To an outsider, especially such an outsider as Vin, Skip's new boyfriend, who would be motivated to condemn the relationship, it would appear to be just the simple transaction that is called prostitution.

Neither Skip nor I thought of our relationship as prostitution, but there *was* money in it and a strong whiff of sex, though not sex itself. Consequently both felt the steady threat of the simpler conceptualization, a steady threat to self-esteem and the need to believe that "he is not with me for money alone" and "he does not value me out of lust alone." Our relationship would have been cleaner and simpler if it had been one of prostitution. The ambiguities would have been eliminated, as well as all of the psychological interest.

I mailed my letter late at night and regretted it first thing in the morning. It was a disastrous letter! Skip knew it all already and my weakness was revolting. But a letter, once mailed, belongs to the U.S. Postal Service. It was still in the building, in the mailbox in the hall. Was there any way to retrieve it? I remembered that Jack, the security guard on duty, used to be the mailman.

"Jack, I mailed a letter last night and by mistake used the wrong address. Is there any way to get it back?"

"Sure, I'll ask George to fish it out when he opens the box."

Whew!

* * *

I still did not know about Vin, but I knew I was losing Skip. I decided to make one last try. On Friday, January 17, I called.

"I'm calling to invite you to go with me for five days to St. Bart's in the Caribbean. I've never been there, but they say it's the most beautiful island. It's French, and you'd have to get a passport."

"Wow, a passport! It sounds great but I doubt I can go."

"Why not? You'd only miss a couple of days at work. I would rent a villa right on the beach and, of course, we'd have separate bedrooms and bathrooms. I thought I'd rent a jeep too and we could tool around the island from one beach to another." I could not have said where I learned the verb "to tool" or picked up the knowledge that young people think jeeps are cool.

"I don't know."

"Will you come over for one whole evening and talk about the possibility?'"

A long pause, and then a hissing, existential "Yesss. But I can't see you until Monday, the twentieth. I . . . I'm going out of town for a couple of days."

A three-day delay. Skip *never* went out of town; he didn't even have a car. "I know what that means. You're dated up with someone and can't get away. More deceit? More lies! I can't go back to that!"

"What's *wrong* with you? I think you're a schizophrenic. One minute you're all sweet talk and the next you're calling me a liar. Okay, I'm not going out of town. I'll explain when I see you."

On Monday, the twentieth, Skip told the tale of Vin—or some of it. Skip's theory of personality was that it rose out of ethnicity. "Vin is a big Guido and, naturally, he's passionate and violent. I told him about our friendship but he doesn't understand. He says you're a degenerate and he's forbidden me to see you again. He's also told me I have to give up Jim, my best friend, and Groovy. And I can only go to work out at the gym when he comes along. He's trying to change everything in my life, and I've only known him two weeks. I'm definitely not in love with him. He's trying to turn me into a Stepford wife, and I'm only 25 years old and I've never ever been out of the country. He says if I go on a trip with you I'm out of his life. Well, I'm going."

"Are you sure you should? Trips aren't important. If you're in love with him, forget the trip."

"I'm not. I want to go."

"Well, you'll have to apply for the passport right away; it takes a minimum of a week. I'll see Sheila at World Travel and start making the arrangements."

And the countdown began.

St. Bart's is a very small island. Sheila said one can drive all around it in half a day. Would there be enough to do to keep Skip entertained? He's a very kinetic young man. It seemed there was scuba and surfing, and Skip loved both. Mealtimes might be a problem. The two of us were not good at long conversations. We might meet people but there was no gay life at all on St. Bart's.

Skip had his own ideas about how we would stay entertained. From Groovy he would get some pot and several hits of ecstasy.

"We're going to an island paradise, Skip, and it sounds as if we have to drug ourselves insensible in order to bear it."

Skip had his own reasons for thinking he might have trouble bearing it. Because of Vin's repeated interdiction and his own strong wish to go, he was crying a lot and not sleeping well and already smoking a lot of pot.

Vin sent me a letter at my office. The printing on the envelope foretold the content; it was all thick, black, bold strokes.

Professor,

Skip informed me of his "friendship" with you. His recounts of your activity in his life were posed as a benign acquaintance. As time went on I learned of how you two met through a professional escort agency in Boston and I was told of the Christmas trip to New York City. Your relationship with and influence on Skip was beginning to smack of unseemly motivation. Red flags raised upon your offering Skip a Caribbean trip which is anguishing him no end to refuse. He also describe to me of your ostensibly hiring him for $500.00 a week as your personal escort.

I realized, at that time, that your relationship was not one based on friendship, but your overwhelming need to have a cute young man by your side, at whatever monetary cost. I am giving Skip an alternative: choose you or me.

Roger, I don't know what you had with your lover. I am sorry he has passed. It is difficult and lonely to be young and gay. I can only imagine where the loss of a life long companion leaves you. Your desperation for company is evident.

You are an old, tired faggot, Professor. The type of person who makes being gay unattractive and difficult. You prey on the young maladjusted with your financial propositions and further perpetuate an already abject cycle.

Vin

With this letter, my entire history with Skip did a perceptual flip-flop. I saw perfectly Vin's point of view and despised myself for the role I had played. But Skip totally repudiated Vin's version. I had known Skip for six months before Vin came on the scene. Skip had been a callboy long before I met him and thanks to me and my friends had developed the self-esteem to give it up. In any case, Boston Dream Boys were nothing like the maladjusted youths Vin imagined. I had never asked Skip to have sex with me and the salary I paid had had no strings attached but was intended to make Skip's life a little easier, etc. I was able to see my own point of view once more and banish Vin's, at least temporarily.

Skip asserted that his intention to make the trip was steadfast, but he was obviously under great nervous strain. Hoping to divert him, I took Skip to visit Sue and Peg, the couple he liked so much, with their two cats, whom Skip loved as much as the ladies. Before going I told Skip to feel free to talk about Vin and about his quandary. He did talk about Vin, starting with his bossiness and violence and other faults but, as he talked, I noticed an evaluative drift in the content to Vin's good looks, passionate lovemaking, and basic brilliance. Sue and Peg, listening to what had become a paean of praise, were horribly embarrassed, but I seemed scarcely to mind.

Outside it was bitter cold and there was a coating of ice on the street. Skip was going to Groovy's house in Porter Square, five miles out of my way. The old man was not a very good driver and ought not to have insisted on driving Skip to his destination.

"You be very careful, puddin'. I'm going to call you to make sure you get home safely."

I did get home safely and in good time but the phone did not ring all night. Next day Skip said: "I called but there was no answer. I guess it was before you got home." I could not find comfort in this explanation.

The day before the trip Skip called in the morning: "My passport came and I'm all packed. I'm *excited!*"

About four he called again and with absolute finality said: "Roger, honey, I can't go."

Chapter 6

Grant

What is the best prediction to make of someone's social behavior? Repetition. The same thing as before. Is this true even when it has turned out badly, as my courtship of Skip did? Even then. Perhaps especially then. Freud called it "repetition compulsion," the compulsion to repeat styles of action, even total relationships that can never have given pleasure. Among his examples are the benefactor whose protégés always turn against him and the lover whose love affairs all pass through the same dismal phases. The impression such people give, Freud wrote, "is of being pursued by a malignant fate or some demonic power."

Freud wrote as if the compulsion to repeat operated on the total relationship or cycle of action, but that is not the way it works. I did not choose to be thrown over by the young men I courted or to be made to suffer by their neglect. It was only the first step I felt compelled to take and to repeat: making the effort to win the love of a handsome young man using charm, money, and reputation to compensate for age and its infelicities. What made it look as if I chose to repeat the full pattern was the seeming inevitability of the outcome and so its foreseeability.

My friends, hearing my stories of panic over neglect, angry farewells, repentance, and forgiveness, interpreted these repetitions in Freud's way and gently suggested that I *created* these lovers' crises to keep passion alive. But it was not so. I hated the disappointments and panics; my suffering was real. I could see ahead to the inevitable bad outcomes but was not convinced of their absolute inevitability. What I chose to repeat was not a doomed enterprise but a very high-risk enterprise, an assault on Mount Everest. And, having failed to attain Mount Everest, which is what Skip was, I did not let that rule out a more foolhardy enterprise soon to present itself: a shot at the moon.

When Skippy decided he could not go to St. Bart's, my life ought to have ended. Ours had been a great romance, climaxing in a great conflict; a decisive choice had been made and a good curtain line delivered. I felt the dramatic necessity of passing on and did manage to get quite sick—sick enough to cause one doctor to suspect a recurrence of prostatic cancer—but then I passed a large kidney stone and immediately felt quite a lot better.

Skippy and I never having been lovers, I had recourse to the occasional Dream Boy throughout the entire affair and, the narcissistic wounds inflicted by Skippy being what they were, I had hoped to meet a d.b. appealing enough to start a flame in my heart as backfire, so to speak, to the raging conflagration set by Skip. This had not happened. However, some ten days after the St. Barthélemy Massacre, Bruce, of Dream Boys, intruded on my despair with an interesting call.

"I think we have someone you'd be interested in meeting. His name's Grant, and he says he's on a sabbatical from the University of Michigan."

"Sabbatical? *I'm* on sabbatical. Only professors get sabbaticals—are you sure he said 'sabbatical'?"

"That's what he said. I don't even *know* what a sabbatical is, but he doesn't look like a professor. What he looks like is a football player. He's older than most of our boys, but he has . . . *compensating qualities.*" This last was said with that "if you know what I mean" insinuation which, in Bruce, substituted for knowledge of the arts and sciences. "He's studying to be a doctor, and I thought you, being a doctor at the university, might like to meet him."

"I guess I would—just out of curiosity."

Bruce's grid of categories for persons was coarse-grained, and in that grid Grant probably looked more like a football player than anything else. He was over six feet tall, with immense shoulders, deep-chested with huge hands but elegant, not burly, and with a straight-arrow face. His dark hair was stubble short and smelled like fresh-cut clover. A Kevin Costner look-alike, he was everyone's vision of a truly handsome and decent man and, therefore, like no d.b. that ever lived.

"Yo," in a deep voice that broke a little as he shifted registers from manly to friendly.

Grant and I sat side by side on the leather couch and I did the talking, the whole story of Skip through the dumping ten days ago. Grant, in telling Bruce that he was on sabbatical, had assumed that in Boston, the city of universities, anyone would understand his usage was jocular. What he meant was he had interrupted his pre-med studies to take a look around and see whether medicine was really what he wanted. For starters he was doing a six-week apprenticeship in publishing (unpaid) with the Harvard University Press.

"I guess, feeling as bad as you do about your friend Skip, you don't feel like fooling around."

Fooling around? thought I. Is it possible that this is this guy's way of talking about sex? Fooling around? Snapping towels at one another in the locker room? I had not felt so feminized since I put my feet up in stirrups so they could biopsy the prostate. I did not feel up to shaking hands, let alone "fooling around."

"I'm going back to the Upper Peninsula to go hunting and fishing with my friend Hank. I'll send you a card."

And a card did come, sent, I calculated, on the last day of the Michigan trip. The card read: "Bet you didn't think I'd send a card." I was once again at the Ritz-Carlton for milieu therapy when Grant reappeared. And what a reappearance! He came striding down the hall, carrying a dozen three-foot white gladiolus—Cary Grant come to court Katharine Hepburn.

"Don't make anything out of the flowers. Since you were feeling so bad last time—"

On this visit I did feel like fooling around, and the room at the Ritz had a big bed with a facing TV screen. I undertook to interest Grant in the superior qualities of the pornography of Jean-Daniel Cadinot. Cadinot made good use of reaction shots so one knew what a given operation *felt* like, not simply how it was *executed*. Grant was in fact aroused by the Cadinot video, and when he reached orgasm it was like a locomotive pulling into Grand Central Station; Grant shook, I shook, the chandelier shook. And afterwards:

"I'm gonna jump in the shower."

"Of course, you *jump* into the hot shower, I think I'll just slip into a warm tub."

"There is that difference between you and me, isn't there?"

I laughed. "Not really, but I can tell you'd like to think so."

Grant was sexually very exciting to me. Sometimes I would have an erection, not something that would cut glass but very serviceable. Pressing it with some pride against Grant's butt, I would be told, "Don't *even* think about it. Don't *even* think about it."

I wanted to have sex far more often than Grant did. I was not supposed to take this asymmetry seriously; it had been true of all Grant's lovers, women as well as men, and their numbers had been roughly equal.

"Sex just isn't important to me." This from the man who, above all others, had been specifically designed by God to give erotic satisfaction.

It was not as a source of erotic satisfaction that I interested Grant; it was as a man of learning, a scholar, and a wit. "I respect you. You've accomplished things. You make me laugh."

On Grant's first visit I brought out the copy of *Harvard Magazine* with a picture of me and a cute tyke on the cover, and inside a flattering story about my work called "How Children Learn Language." This instrument of seduction, when sprung on Skip, got "Holy shit!" and nothing more. But Grant read the article–most of it on the spot–and it fathered the concept of a series of paperback books for parents on aspects of cognitive development in childhood. And Grant should be the series editor in chief, with me as individual editor of one volume.

Grant was so excited about his idea that he overstayed his time; the $220 Dream Boy was for one hour and a half. When Bruce called to find out what was up, Grant told him to fuck off. Bruce, unaccustomed to so much testosterone, just shut up.

At first, I tried to match Grant's level of enthusiasm for the projected series on cognitive development. I could not tell him the idea was not new; just such a series had been brought out by another publisher and was doing well.

Grant took his inspiration to the director of the Harvard University Press and the director seemed to Grant so enthusiastic that Grant feared his idea might be stolen. When nothing at all came of it and he stopped returning Grant's calls, I guessed that the director, like myself, had found the enthusiasm of the vital young man irresistible but counted on Grant's follow-through to wise him up to the problems.

But there was no follow-through. There never was follow-through on Grant's projects. He believed that an inspired idea could directly create a great success without hard work. Grant had a store of projects, and, sooner or later, one of them would pay off.

When I realized that Grant's thinking was hopelessly magical, I worked hard to protect the young man from that knowledge. My heart ached because it seemed likely that the dream of an inspired *strike* accounted for the fact that so appealing a man was still bouncing around with no vocation.

Publishing as a career ended with his six-week apprenticeship at Harvard University Press. Unaware that the apprenticeship was over, I called Grant at work.

"Grant Flag? Anybody here know a Grant Flag? Oh, the intern. He's long gone."

I wondered how Grant was living. The young man's fierce independence made it impossible to ask, but several things were incidentally divulged. He was on call as a substitute teacher in the Boston schools but had become choosy about assignments after a single day of riot control duty. Some weekends he worked as a helper on a construction job. Escorting? Probably not, as he hated it and only tried it out of desperation.

"I'd like to put you on a retainer of $500 a week so you can get out of Dream Boys and stabilize yourself."

"I'll have to think about it."

Ten days later: "You still want an answer on your offer?"

"Of course."

"The answer is okay, but on condition it doesn't affect our relationship."

When Grant first arrived in Boston, he was immediately taken up by what he called the "A set"–the best-looking young gay men. I felt sure he must have been their brightest star. I once told Rebecca, "Grant is quite simply the handsomest gay man I've ever seen. You'll have trouble believing he is gay; and in fact he's not; he's bisexual in a gay phase."

I had, before this, heard talk of "A," "B," and "C" sets of gay men and lesbians. What the qualifications were, how they "dated" and "married" selectively, each set practicing homogamy. It was comical to see the excitement with which these nonacademic young people "discovered" social structure. Once, in a mean mood, I told several of them about the sociological classic "The Rating and Dating Complex," by William Waller, which describes "A," "B," and "C" classes in American fraternities in the 1930s. Ratings those days depended on looks, clothes, dancing, cars, and, for all we know, breasts and penises. Supremely well-qualified for the "As," Grant had, just before he met me, turned his back on them.

"All they're interested in is drinking, and doing drugs, partying." Like Coriolanus in Rome, Grant knew there was "a world elsewhere," and he banished the A set forever. When one or another A's spoke to him in the gym he did not even reply. Now he found me and Jack Quilty and a few others much more congenial.

Grant had dropped his premedical studies and his friends at Michigan; he dropped the A set and, I learned, an A-rated boyfriend. Recently he had dropped publishing, though he still spoke wistfully about his projects.

Jack Quilty's formulation was that Grant habituated fast. "Habituated" is a psychological term for getting used to something to the point where it becomes predictable and uninteresting. The formulation was consistent with Grant's thinking. There was just one thing, so far as I knew, that did not fit. Grant, an out-of-state applicant, had been admitted to the University of Michigan and so must have had excellent high school grades, and he had earned honors grades in the difficult courses of the premed program. Therefore in earlier years, in high school and college at least, he must have worked and controlled any tendency to habituate. There was a mysterious discontinuity of character between Grant-as-student and Grant-in-Boston.

What no one knew was that, about a year earlier, when he made the decision to take a sabbatical, Grant started to think he might be HIV positive. But he did not get tested. What he knew was that Marius Malleis, who had been his lover for three months in Paris, now had AIDS. Grant, like many others who think they might be seropositive, chose not to know, because not knowing made it possible much of the time not to think about it.

Not knowing his HIV status also made it possible for Grant to *work at* making it negative. He did this by making himself look and feel like a young god—someone who could not be seropositive, let alone someone who could have AIDS.

Grant's diet was designed to produce muscle: protein shakes and no greasy foods. He worked out two hours a day with a trainer to see he did things right. Many young gay men work out on a similarly arduous schedule today, and gay men of earlier generations, who remember hating gym class, are sometimes surprised. The difference is that "working out" links strenuous exercise with narcissism instead of team competition, and also often with sexual contacts.

In a large city there will be one or more gay gyms where attractive men make out like gangbusters. Grant despised such places and went only to gyms that were strictly heterosexual. Any homosexual element that got into Grant's life had to get past his heterosexual guard, by either by wearing a disguise or taking him by surprise.

Skip once asked me: "What's Grant got that I haven't?"

"It isn't that he has got anything more or even that he's more attractive to me. The difference is, he seems to like me better. For one thing, he is interested in my work and admires me for it. I can be myself with him and don't have to enter a hopeless competition with cool kids." That was as much as I chose to tell Skip, but there was more to it.

The great thing was that Grant had sex with me: not just Skippy-play but sex and orgasm. The active parts were all played by Roger, but I took it for granted it had to be that way at my hard-luck age. Skip was wonderful at petting but shrank from anything more, as if my body made him uneasy.

After the first half-dozen times, I had to tug the pants off Grant, fighting his considerable dead weight. Grant was nevertheless easily aroused and quick to climax. I did not mind the friendly uncooperativeness because I came to believe Grant's considerable investment in heterosexuality made it necessary for him to show scant enthusiasm, to be passively "serviced" (as a straight man might also be). One time, with unusual candor, Grant said: "You put up with it because you know it's the only way we can do it." Surprisingly, even this very limited acceptance of my body by my young beloved—even these one-sided genital events—made me happier and

more content than I had been with Skip. That is what was meant by
the remark: "He seems to like me better."

Very early on Grant told me his worry about his HIV status and
asked me if I thought we were being safe.

"Yes, I do."

"What makes you think so? Because you want to?"

"Yes, and because I don't care. My life expectancy is about the
same, positive or negative."

"That's true. What would you do if I got sick?"

"I would look after you."

"Even if I didn't want you to. Right?"

"Right. But I want you to get tested. I have had worries like
yours and then got tested—twice—and turned out to be negative. You
have to get tested, not just because there is now an advantage in
early knowledge if you *are* positive, but because your uncertainty is
messing up your life in ways you are not aware of."

I thought Grant's uncertainty helped to explain his recent pattern
of short-term enthusiasms and rejections. In a wave of optimism
about his health status he would take up a new career, new friends,
and a new conception of himself. Any failure, however minor,
reminded him that, if his HIV status were positive, nothing mattered
anyway and he might as well stop trying and drop everything and
everyone.

"Call me as soon as they give you the result."

"Okay, but if it's bad I'm not going to talk about it."

Later: "Yo." The voice on the phone, desolate. "Well, I'm positive."

"Oh, God." So young, so handsome, so fastidious. I knew Grant
must hate getting a disease associated with anal sex, with feminized
"bottoms," with Castro clones, camp, and everything he despised.

"You can start AZT right away and probably have ten years
without symptoms."

"I may have been positive awhile; some of those years may be
used up."

"But you don't know. You're spectacularly healthy. If anyone's
going to beat it, you will."

"Oh, there's always hope. I don't want to talk about it anymore
now." He never talked about it again. He signed up for an exper-

imental treatment program at the Beth Israel Hospital; it meant he got his medications free. When I would ask what they did on any given appointment, the answer would be: "Poking and prodding—forget it." He thought of writing to his parents, to prepare them, but somehow did not and never said anything at all to them about it.

When Grant's T-cell count dropped to the 400 level, the level where opportunistic infections become likely, Jack tried to reassure him by telling him he had a symptom-free friend who had a T-cell count of zero. Grant resented Jack's attempts to play the medical man: "I know more about it than Jack does."

Once in a great while something broke through his Roman stoicism. After a visit to his friend Tom, who was in Beth Israel, Grant said: "His skin is all gray. I'll never get like that. I'll kill myself." Once his control really failed, and when that happened it was so terrible that I had to be grateful for Grant's usual inexpressiveness. On a vacation in San Francisco, fairly late at night, in the suite I shared with Grant, I was building up a steamhead of anger that Grant had not yet shown up, when I heard a sound in the next room: "I don't want to die. I don't want to die." And suddenly Grant, stronger and tougher than anyone I knew, was crying convulsively.

"I saw this girl at a bar. Nothing special, really, but she came on to me big. I wasn't interested but I thought, what if I were, what could I do now?"

When Grant apologized next morning, I said, "I didn't mind. It was humanizing."

"So now you know I'm human."

I did not think about any danger to my own health. Neither did Grant. In fact, encouraged by Grant to believe that he was not having, and did not want, any sex other than the rather tame things the two of us did, I thought Grant's seropositive status was probably what constrained him. "Believe what you want to believe, that's one thing you're good at," Albert had taunted me when I looked away from his impending death.

After the news we had some sad weeks. One morning I called: "Let's go somewhere. Let's see something. There's a new Ritz Hotel in Naples, Florida. I've noticed their ads in *The New Yorker*. Henry Ginger, my new travel agent, says Naples is the class act in Florida. We could leave Saturday morning."

"I'm in the same mood. Let's do it."

"I am really crazy about you, you know."

"I know."

Returned from Naples, in the taxi in Boston, I said to Grant: "I've had one of the best times of my life."

"Really?" Not superciliously, but a little surprised, not able to go that far himself. Grant partially made up for the hurt by gathering my hands in his big mitts and saying: "Thank you for a wonderful, wonderful time."

Some days later, I told Grant that the best moment of the Naples trip had been Grant's taking my hands in the taxi. If Grant had asked why, the explanation would have been the same as one I had given to Kevin in the Touchy-Feely Room eighteen months ago: "Because it's you doing something and not just me."

The impact of Grant's action shows how rare it was for him to express affection. He was the same in speech as in touch. In late-night phone calls he listened politely to my extravagant declarations of love and lavish use of endearments but never let them coerce a reciprocal response. No "Me too" or "I feel the same." The most Grant would do was lay on a warm overtone in saying "Good night." It almost seemed a principle. He was a bit like the title of a certain pornographic movie: *Don't Kiss Me, I'm Straight.*

Grant was a lot like Albert as a lover and the opposite of Skip, at least as Skip was with me. I very much missed Skip's nonverbal tenderness, but Grant's laconic style had its own power. As I had with Albert so many years ago, I got caught up in the challenge of eliciting affection from an inexpressive person. When I got it, the reward was almost enough to make up for the long, dry periods.

Grant, like Albert, was aware of his style and defended it.

"People who talk a lot about how much they love you aren't as reliable when it comes down to it as the quiet ones."

Grant, unlike Roger or Albert, was an outdoor person and a sportsman. He liked backpacking, horseback riding, and boating. He had taught scuba diving in Hawaii. He liked wilderness, jungle, desert, the outback, not civilization. The luxuries of the Naples Ritz meant little to him. The Everglades and the 10,000 islands off the Gulf coast meant a lot; plants and animals and fish and birds were what he cared for. Most of all, he once told me, he would like to have been, necessarily in another age, an explorer. It would be difficult to conceive of an adult personality less like mine, but Grant reminded me of my childhood and, as a boy, I had wanted to be an adventurer, not a pedagogue and a pedophile.

We took a canoe into the Everglades, as far as we could go and come back the same day. Grant paddled while I sat very still in the middle seat. Grant called attention to an osprey nest with young ones in it ("Aren't they neat?") and Grant climbed into an over-hanging tree to tear out a bromeliad plant ("Isn't it cool?") to smuggle onto the plane and bring back to his apartment. I watched with admiration. And the archetypal Everglades look, a tunnel of trees and vines, gave me a boy's thrill of adventure.

Another day we rented a motorboat early in the morning and sampled some of the 10,000 islands and atolls. Again Grant had all the skills and knowledge, knew how to find channels and read ocean depths from ocean colors. He revved up the engine and made the boat spank on the water to give me a thrill. And I was thrilled, by the way the captain looked as well as by his seamanship. When Grant handed me the steering wheel of the speeding boat I tried hard not to be either old or a sissy. Even though I knew myself to be both, it was not painful, because Grant seemed to think I tran-scended such things.

The days on the beach were great. Grant, like me, loved to bake in the sun, and he had his bodybuilding and scuba diving so that we were not too much together. The best time was lunch in an outdoor seafood place, our two pairs of very long legs and very big feet up on the wooden railings, both too sunblasted to do anything but eat and smile at one another. There were also two late afternoons when we tumbled into bed together in the air-conditioned dark, and there are no words adequate to those afternoons.

Dinners were awkward because service was slow in the fancy places we went, and much conversation had to be made. At the last dinner I asked Grant how it happened that a Montana cowpoke used his knife and fork in the Continental style. That stimulated Grant to set me straight on his background. His folks had been and were poor, but they kept horses and he learned to play polo as well as to bulldog steers. Polo players were mostly rich, and so Grant had expensive tastes and plenty of sophistication, more really than I, for whom the chain of Ritz hotels seemed the dernier cri, and Grant said "dernier cri " with, to be sure, a vile accent.

When we said "good night" at our respective bedroom doors, Grant felt confident enough to say something funny and a little bit feminine: "Thanks for dinner." As if he were a little number apologizing for not coming across at the end of an expensive evening. For both of us this became a permanent memory, a flashbulb fired by feeling, still in the future but presaged in that moment.

With Skip, I had said: "You'll miss me when I'm gone." I had always realized that the strain between us must eventually separate us and that it would be me, Roger, who would make the break, because it was I who felt the greater discomfort.

With Grant, I would say: "I don't see any reason why we shouldn't always be friends, since each of us is being himself." To Grant I said on the phone one Saturday morning: "I have a deep feeling of well-being, of happiness, today and the only reason I can think of is that you're in my life."

Grant never made remarks like these, but then it was part of Grant's style as a man's man to be laconic.

"It's my dad who made such a big deal out of my being a man's man. I remember when I was little him telling a neighbor: 'He's all man; we saw to that.'"

And was he not, I reflected. Very strong, very good at horseback riding, boating, football, carpentry, woodsmanship, and car repairs. He was even homophobic; he couldn't stand effeminacy or camp. Was there anything at all about him that was not perfectly manly?

Once when we were out shopping for sport shirts, standing behind Grant I caught him striking a pose for the mirror that was clearly intended to be a cowboy leaning on a bar. Getting in and out of boats, Grant was perhaps unnecessarily reckless and disdainful of any helping hand. Walking with me, Grant did not at all accommodate his titanic stride to my older-man's pace. Automobiles he drove expressively, with plenty of screeching tires and changing of lanes. Noting these slight excesses, Barry once said there was something histrionic about Grant's style. Did he perhaps feel that he was acting? In Grant's adult manliness a slight excess was the only flaw one could detect.

When Grant was eleven years old, back in Montana, his father came upon what he considered a major flaw in his son's manliness. "Me and this other kid were looking at our penises–just out of curiosity. My dad caught us and yelled at me: 'You God-damned little faggot.' Then he beat my face in. You might say that was a memorable lesson."

When Grant grew up, the masculine independence his father had encouraged gave the young man the strength to tell his father: "Accept me as I am or you will never see me again." Grant's mother was included in the challenge, but in this family mother went for very little. For five years now Grant and his father have not seen one another and their few telephone conversations have been limited to business affairs.

* * *

Just two weeks after St. Bart's fell through, Mary Croft, secretary to the superintendent of the apartment building where I lived, left a note under the door: "Skippy hopes you are getting along okay." No one had ever before used Mary Croft as a conduit. She must have been astonished by the novelty of the event, and I did not even know how Skip would have got her number. But how well suited to his purposes the mode of communication was. He did not want to talk to me, to answer any questions or listen to accusations, just to express concern: "You are in my thoughts."

Skip sent messages two more times, and I lamely explained to Mary Croft: "He seems to be very concerned about my health; I'm not sure why." In my own mind I asked: Is there really some residual affection? Is the thing with Vin going sour? Is he asking for a second chance? And I reflected: He doesn't know that I'm now totally concentrated on Grant.

On February 10, the week before Valentine's Day, there came a valentine of unmistakable origin. On a red envelope the return address in the upper left-hand corner was an "S" with a star and, as address, the letters of my name in a variety of fonts interspersed with hearts and flowers. Inside it read: "If I don't see you, Happy Valentine's Day. . . . You are in my thoughts. Hugs to Edwige, Sue, Peg, Jack, Barry, Anthony, and *you*." What most surprised and interested me in this message was the phrase "If I don't see you," which expressed a presupposition that I and my friends might reasonably have expected to see Skip before Valentine's Day. I had no such expectation. When I broke up with someone, I meant to break up forever, and my mind started at once erasing every memory trace. Probably it was an adaptation to years of heavy teaching, when a "preparation," once it was used, had to make room for the next one. In my mind it was irrevocably over. Was it not in Skip's? These days I was not much interested in reading Skip's mind, but I did rather like feeling courted.

The week of March 10-16 Skip spent in Puerto Rico. I thought Puerto Rico would have made a good consolation present from Vin for the forgone St. Bart's, but Skip went with "best friend" Jim. Indeed, I had heard nothing about Vin for two months. Skip sent a card: "Miss talking with you. Hope all is well with you, Edwige, Dr. Quilty, etc." The most characteristic thing on this card was "*Dijo que te amo*" with an attached obliterating "Not." Skip had always liked to come close to saying "I love you," always taking care to say that it was not so to anyone who might take it seriously. For this romantic young man, the phrase "I love you" was a serious one; he had never said it to me.

On March 20, just four days after returning from Puerto Rico and seven weeks after saying "no" to St. Bart's, Skip called to say that Vin had hit him and so was definitely being terminated. Skip, having seen his father beat up his mother, could not tolerate violence. He was dismayed to hear about Grant and wanted to see me for a full evening in order to explain some things I had not correctly understood.

"I'm glad about Grant and hope he is making you happy. You can tell him from me that he has a wonderful man."

Always glad of any endorsement, I did pass on these remarks to Grant but was disappointed in the reaction.

"A typical bitchy gay effort to make trouble. Just what I can't stand."

Why couldn't Grant, I thought, have given the easy Lana Turner answer: "I *know* I've got a wonderful man and I *intend* to make him happy." That line was not in Grant's repertoire.

"I'd like to see Skip, but since he was your predecessor I think I should ask if it's okay with you."

Grant snorted: "I have no predecessor! You know better than to ask me something like this!" No trace of jealousy.

Grant was, in general, rather unpleasantly superior about Skippy. Once, when Skip and I had had dinner, Grant asked: "How was the conversation?" I was quick enough and loyal enough to say: "The conversation was only fair but the communication was perfect."

Skip did not get to meet Grant. He wanted to, but Grant declined, on the grounds that Skip in no way interested him. "Besides, I don't like the way he treated you."

* * *

As a psychologist, in all the years before Skippy and Grant, I had thought individual differences in personality were exaggerated. I compared personality psychologists to cultural anthropologists who took pleasure in, and indeed derived status from, the exoticism of their discoveries. I had once presumed to say to Henry A. Murray, Harvard's distinguished personologist: "I think people are all very much the same."

Murray's response had been: "Oh you do, do you? Well, you don't know what the hell you're talking about!" And I hadn't. My intimates, all my professional life, had been middle-class intellectuals my own age, and one might say of *this* cohort that they were pretty much alike. They had certainly not prepared me to understand Michael Broad, the charming cultivated jewel thief.

Nor had they prepared me for Skippy and Grant. And Skippy turned out to be the worst possible propaedeutic to understanding Grant. But, because the two played the same role in my life—the young beloved—I started out transferring to Grant interpretations better suited to Skip. After five months of these, it is not surprising that Grant, in exasperation, said: "I don't think you understand anything at all about me."

The hierarchy of Grant's interests exactly reversed Skip's. First came his work; second came boating, horseback riding, scuba diving—large-muscle, outdoor pleasures, with animals or machines; social relationships trailed badly, and love and sex were last. I, ever the suitor, had to retrain my selective memory. At first I would forget Grant's publishing projects or the people involved and would be told: "You have to *listen* to me. Is this a good idea or not? I want your serious opinion." Or I would make the kind of joke about sex that Skip used to enjoy and Grant would say: "I don't care about that. *Teach* me something. I like to learn."

The most unfortunate effect of my experience with Skip on my interpretation of Grant was the attribution to Grant of Skip's deceit in connection with Vin and with less important lovers.

One Saturday, Grant had invited Jack and me to lunch and was to call before noon to specify restaurant and time. Jack and I waited together until almost two and then called. Grant answered the phone in a groggy voice: "I jus' need a li'l more sleep."

That was enough to create the most florid suspicions in my mind and Jack, being very much amused by my operatic jealousies, said nothing to calm them and, indeed, pointed up possible parallels to Skippy. Since Grant still needed more sleep in the afternoon, I supposed that he had been out all night. His voice suggested he'd been drinking and perhaps doing drugs. It was easy to imagine him stumbling around in his apartment, stepping over some naked trick, unconscious on the futon. Jack's contribution was: "I never did buy that story about his low sex drive; you only need to look at the guy. For all you know he has another boyfriend, a real one."

The truth is that when Grant entered our lives, Jack could no longer be the unselfish, even solicitous friend to me that he used to be and still pretended to be because, not to insist on a fresh phrase when the right one has been coined, he fell for Grant like a ton of bricks. It was Jack who most successfully hit upon Grant's special appeal: "He's the most glamorous man I ever met." "Glamorous" is a word that can be aptly used of a movie star or an explorer, suggesting as it does not only attraction but also adventure, excitement, and magic; for Grant it was the right word.

Grant liked Jack and flirted with him and may even have preferred his company to mine. In any case, he seemed better pleased by the prospect of a social threesome than an evening of hanging out alone with the horny professor; but that may just have been his distaste for everlasting erotic pursuit. The result of all this was that Jack's interpretation of Grant became sly and self-serving and confirmed my fears and suspicions. It was some time before I noticed this.

As we walked to lunch I hit my head with my fists: "Once, yes. It could happen once to anybody. But twice, and in immediate succession; how could I be so gullible?" But it was not so. Grant was not guilty of the things attributed to him. He had been unable to sleep all night and toward dawn had taken two Halcion pills that someone had given him. He was susceptible to Halcion and probably to all sleeping pills, since he never took any. The pills had knocked him out for hours and Grant threw into the toilet the few he had left: "Those things are poison."

To me, Grant explained the difference between himself and Skip, patiently the first time but angrily at last when I seemed unable to learn. "When I foul up, and I'm bound to sometimes, it's never going to be because of sex. I'm just not interested in sex with strangers or in starting a romance. I can always find them. They're always being offered to me. But I really don't want them. I like you; can't I convince you of that? I respect you and you make me laugh. All my friends are handsome. What does handsome do for me?"

I was slow in learning about people, but I did eventually realize that Grant was completely trustworthy: no lies, no deceit, nothing on the side. He deserved his straight-arrow face. I was in a good position to see the value of trustworthiness; it relieved me of the demeaning and exhausting business of playing detective and interrogator. Jack seemed eager to do it for me.

* * *

The flight back from Naples was one of the happiest times I ever spent with Grant—until, that is, Grant went over some papers and recollected a certain problem. Both of us looked great with fresh tans and dressed, coincidentally, in Cambridge uniform: khaki trousers, blindingly white shirts, navy-blue blazers, and "power" neckties (red and yellow). Handsome father and handsomer son, the flight attendants took us for. And Grant capped my bliss by saying: "I like the way we look together."

The papers Grant took from his elegant attaché case in the last hour of the flight concerned a lawsuit to be held in Ann Arbor two days thence. Grant's father, on Grant's urging, had purchased a certain house in Ann Arbor which Grant had rented, injudiciously as it turned out, to three students who proved to be hooligans and did a lot of damage. Grant, on his father's behalf, was suing for damages. But now, on the plane back from Naples, Grant read the

fine print requiring him to obtain and file certain depositions prov-
ing that the house was in fact damaged by the former tenants. He
had put the responsibility out of his mind, and now it was too late.
Grant and his father would certainly lose the lawsuit.

The negligence, not Grant's first, unstoppered a great store of
guilt. Grant figured he owed his father; in the first place, he wasn't
the son the stupid man wanted. I interpolated: "If I had a son, I can't
imagine anyone more ideal than you." If he could not be the son his
father wanted, and he could not, Grant thought at least he might have
stayed at Michigan in his premed program as his father wished.

Unable to satisfy these wishes, Grant could not stand to cost the
poor man money, but that was now going to happen. The Ann Arbor
house was up for sale but would never sell unless the damage was
repaired, but repairs would cost money that neither father nor son
had. The damages from the lawsuit would have done that.

"I'll just have to fix the house myself. I know how, but it means
spending the summer in Ann Arbor. And I don't know how I can do
that, since I won't be working at a job that brings in any income.
What a mess! Well, I'll work it out somehow."

My heart just about stopped beating. Grant absent all summer! I
had a fatalistic feeling that it would be my last summer in good-
enough health to be enjoyed. Grant was the centerpiece of this
conception. Without him the summer dried up and died.

Grant's problems could be solved with money. It would take
quite a lot of money, but I was willing. The problem was going to be
Grant; how could he be persuaded to accept a large sum of money?

I thought of a way to make what I roguishly called my Faustian
Proposition. "Faustian" by loose analogy with Mephistopheles'
offer: "In this life I will be at your service but afterwards you will
be at mine."

It was not exactly Grant's soul I hoped to buy. What was it, then?
His ass? That would be great, but it was not the essential thing. Was
it just his occasional company? More than that. Surely not his love!
I would buy it if I could, but I knew no sum could do that.

No, it was just enough attention—phone calls, acceptance of invitations, thoughtful gifts—to support me in a feeling of—not love—
but great affection, freedom from being undeceived, as it were. Not
a lot from my point of view. What I overlooked, as did Grant at first,

was the fact that satisfying Roger's wishes meant surrendering some freedom, by a man whose life was guided by the principle: "I never do anything I don't want."

On June 6, a U.S. Treasury note in my portfolio would mature and its value was $30,000. I had decided after Al's death had ceased to engulf my mind and I had a chance to check out my retirement funds, to consolidate my assets, think about my likely life span, and face the fact that I did not care much about enriching any of my relatives. I had decided, after all that, that I had no interest in increasing my equity and so would try to spend all my income and gradually reduce my capital. My goal was to spend my last penny as I drew my last breath—"a neat trick not easily managed," my great friend in psychology, Stanley Milgran, had commented. The $30,000 meant nothing to me and its marginal utility, if that is the right concept, compared to Grant's presence in Cambridge was zero. Why not therefore give the $30,000 to Grant to solve all the problems that called him to Ann Arbor?

To my surprise, Grant did not simply dismiss the proposal with a laugh. He listened to my reasons and reflected. He pointed out I would be sacrificing the interest on the $30,000, that interest was income, not capital.

"But it would only come to about $2,000 a year, and that's an insignificant amount."

Grant understood my lack of interest in enriching relatives; he felt the same way himself.

"Tell me again, Roger, why you want me to have this money."

"There are unselfish reasons, such as I don't think you should be wasting your talents on manual labor at this time in your life, and I don't think your father should allow you to. The main reason, however, is selfish. I love your company and would miss you terribly."

"You could always visit weekends."

"In theory, yes, but Ann Arbor is a difficult place to get to. I doubt it would work out."

"What you're saying is it's a completely selfish offer. I'd be doing you a favor. Does that make sense?"

"Yes."

"And there are no strings attached?"

"None."

"You do understand that I am a very independent person. I don't do anything I don't want to do and I don't accept any limits anybody wants to put on me."

"I understand and I've seen that it is the case."

"Then I accept. Thank you."

In spite of my persuasive reasons, I was taken aback by the acceptance. I once offered to lend, not give, a former graduate student $10,000 to meet a pressing obligation. The man just laughed: "I don't want to owe you." There was something about Grant's acceptance that did not fit my picture. Having worked hard to get the gift accepted, my thoughts were unfairly reversed: "You just don't *do* that." Of course I did not say it.

I was completely sincere in agreeing to the "no strings attached" provision; but then what are "strings"? I was assuming that Grant's wishes would continue as they were now, that he would always wish to telephone me daily, to see me a couple of times a week, and to have sex with me about once a week. All this was just fine. Therefore "no strings attached" posed no threat.

In time, however, Grant came to wish to do things that entailed seeing less of me and to talk less often on the telephone. His former practices came to feel like strings, and for me to insist was unfair. To me the practices seemed not to be strings, so it would have been fair under the contract to insist.

I never did straightforwardly insist on certain phone calls on a certain amount of Grant's time and expressions of affection. Instead I got angry and resentful at what I felt were unjust violations, violations—by neglect or omission. The sovereign cause of anger is frustration perceived as unjust. When you do everything right and on time and do not get what you are entitled to—whether it is as important as a promotion or as trivial as catching a bus—you feel anger. That came to be my chronic state of mind, concealed most of the time but sometimes erupting in a verbal jab.

A second powerful cause of anger is to be attacked unjustly. That is what happened to Grant, and he would not put up with it. And so this Faustian Contract was guaranteed to drive apart the two men who agreed to it.

By early July, Grant had had about as much as he could tolerate of me and went off to the Florida Everglades to visit his friend

Amanda; he did not trouble to say for how long. After three days, though no call was scheduled, it was reasonable to expect one as humanitarian relief to me. None came and one evening after too much to drink I left this message: "Three days have gone by and I have not heard a word from you. That is because *you are a cold-hearted son of a bitch.*"

When I was angry I would forget all about Grant's HIV status, but when I cooled off I would remember and be deeply remorseful. It was easy to forget, because Grant looked completely well, easy for others but not for Grant, I knew, and ought always to have remembered.

One might wonder why I set such store by phone calls. It was because the essential message was not the supposed one but rather a message of reassurance to the old gentleman. Reassurance that this godling, Grant, really could care anything about me.

Grant knew very well that reassurance was the needed message and said so to me and to Jack Quilty. Why, then, did he not deliver it, since its importance to me was so great? It was not that he did not call often. It was just that the demands were too obsessively scheduled and so felt like the strings that the Devil's Contract forbade. In a summarizing Bill of Complaints Grant wrote: "Calling all the time is *not me;* constant contact/affection/reassurance is *not me.*" Independence, he warned me, was his essence.

Grant made other changes and was too independent to allow me any voice in the decisions. I heard about them afterward. Grant hated the inner-city neighborhood of his first Boston apartment. It was a very noisy, drug-dealing, dangerous spot. He had two things stolen from his apartment. One night he was knocked unconscious and very badly beaten up, so badly that there were facial abrasions still visible after six weeks. It was a cabdriver who beat him up, just because he did not have enough money on him to pay the fare. He had been drunk, however, and I could well imagine the high-handed manner that would have caused the driver to jump him from behind.

"I have always lived where it's green. I can't be me in the city."

Grant moved to the town of Newbury, about thirty minutes from Boston, where it was green and pretty and where he could moor his boat, if he had had a boat. I could hardly object to anything so idyllic, but I could not help thinking that Newbury was a lot like

Ann Arbor, the city the Contract had been designed to keep Grant from spending the summer in.

"I think you'll see just as much of me as if I'd stayed in Boston." I very much doubted it.

One Sunday Grant came to pick me up to go to the beach. He stayed outside with the jeep and just sent in a message with the doorman. To me this seemed a maneuver to avoid even a moment of intimacy. Had he come in, there would have been at least a quick squeeze. Presumably Grant was not in the mood.

On the drive Grant said, "Oh, I'm expecting Amanda for a couple of days. She's bringing her daughter, which will be nice. I'll be showing them the sights of Boston and the North Shore."

"Everything seems to be conspiring so that I see less and less of you. Sometimes I feel a bit resentful about the money."

"Resentful! You feel resentful! So do I, and I hate that feeling. I thought there were no strings attached to that agreement, which you admitted was totally selfish. I feel plenty of strings. I can't even invite my oldest friend to see my new place. I *know* you feel resentful. I *feel* your anger all the time. You hate everything I care about!"

When we got back from the beach, having stayed only a short time, I managed to catch Grant's eyes and hold them.

"Grant, please come in for a minute."

"No, I've got to get back."

"Grant, there are some things that can't be resolved by talk."

"No, I'm going."

"Grant, don't do this."

"I'm not doing anything."

"Grant, it will hurt me a lot if you just go off."

"Listen, Roger, you always want things on your own terms. Not this time. I'm going."

On the evening of July 3, Grant was scheduled to have dinner with me at the Ritz. I was once again taking my therapy. By staying at the hotel, I hoped to interest Grant in spending time with me. So far Grant had not come near the hotel, but he had promised.

"I'll definitely come for dinner Thursday."

There was no call all day, and it was seven, which was almost too late. I was in the tub when the phone rang, but the Ritz has phones in bathrooms. I sat naked on the edge of the tub and the cold porcelain, dripping water, the too-bright light all flashbulbed permanently into memory as I listened.

"I am out on Route 128 with the last load of stuff that goes to Newbury. I'm afraid I'm not going to make it for dinner."

(Low moan.) "Grant, that's so disappointing. I've been looking forward to seeing you all day, in fact all week."

"I'm sorry, there's just no way I'm going to leave this stuff in my car over the Fourth of July weekend."

"There have been quite a few of these last-minute cancellations and they're really painful. If this is supposed to be a gentle way of 'kissing me off' I'd rather you just said it flat out."

"Listen, I'm going through a rough time right now. I have a job I hate and a disease I hate. Also I carry a lot of baggage about sex. Am I straight or am I gay? Lately I've felt more comfortable with straight men than with gay men."

"And do you also find sex with women more satisfying than sex with men?"

"Oh, *much* more."

In a final note that Grant wrote he added:

> Retrospect indicates your goal or fantasy was to have me molded into something I'm not—the more that becomes conscious to me, the more I am repelled by the idea. Your resentment of me for having accepted the money is all too clear and further fuels the growing discomfort. You offered the sum without strings, as I recall. Therefore I won't tolerate any attempt by you to use that as leverage. In order to continue spending time together, a new and more comfortable space must be found.

I felt totally and forever dismissed.

* * *

In Bangkok in 1989 when Albert was still alive, I had, as I have said, an epileptic seizure. It was the first one ever. On July 10, soon after Grant's note choosing more "space," a second seizure hit the professor, and its cause remained as mysterious as the first. It seemed likely, my life being what it was, there would always be too many medications and too much stress to settle causality for any calamity that might befall me.

I called my secretary: "Sarah, what time is it?"

"Nine-thirty."

"In the morning or at night?"

"In the morning, of course."

"Sarah, maybe you better come over here and call Dr. Quilty to come when he can. Something's wrong with me."

It was not a severe seizure; I bit my tongue; some muscles that do not ordinarily contract did and would be sore for weeks; bowels and bladder, thank God, held tight. Coming out of it there was at first total amnesia. The recovery from amnesia is an interesting process because things come back, not evenly, but in chunks. People seem to come back in order of emotional centrality.

With Sarah, Edwige, and Dr. Quilty as interested listeners, I gave a running account. The first person recalled was, of course, Albert. The fact that Albert was dead came, cruelly, as a separate item after an interval.

"There's someone else. It's Skip." And because immediately after seizure people are very emotional, my eyes welled up.

Jack found Skip's number and he was there in fifteen minutes. Heedless of Sarah, who didn't know him, he put his arms around the professor's neck and showered kisses on his face.

"I'm not going to the Health Services or a neurologist. It'd be the same as last time. They wouldn't be able to tell anything without a million tests, which I'm not having. I'll soon feel fine; I just need someone to stay with me for a little."

"I can stay all day," Skip volunteered. As the others did have obligations, they all went off, leaving their phone numbers and many adjurations.

* * *

"Have you got a job yet, Skip?"

"No, but my friend Jim helped me to write a good résumé and I'm answering lots of ads. I'll find something."

"You shouldn't have quit until you had something better. Why so reckless?"

"I worked hard and they were paying shit. I did a good job too. I did a lot for morale, for one thing."

"I hope you haven't gone back to Dream Boys."

"I could never go back there. Don't you remember, I cheated on them by cutting out to see someone on my own. My name is mud with Dream Boys. There's a new agency called Joshua's, and I did one call for them because I had to have rent, but never again if I can help it."

"What happened?"

"This was this real pig who likes to service guys and do drugs. I was there at his motel about eight at night, and then they called me when I was asleep and he wants me to come back and bring drugs. In the meantime he's had six other guys. I said: 'No way.'"

"That is pretty ugly. If you get stuck for money, I'll help you."

"I hope *you're* not still seeing d.b.s. It's demeaning; you deserve better."

"I know what I deserve, but getting it is the problem. Grant's dumped me; inevitable, I suppose."

"Oh, honey, I'm sorry."

"I don't think I want any more dream boys. Now that I'm approaching the age of–never mind what age–it's time I gave up wrestling with teenagers."

"I think so. Roger, do you know how long we've known each other?"

"Not exactly, it must be close to nine months."

"August 17 will be a year. I wrote it down in my journal. I gave you three stars out of four. Don't you think it's time you married me?"

"Sure. What would married mean?"

"I want to look after you. You need someone. I should move to Cambridge; Dorchester is half an hour away. I'm going to get a beeper and only you'll have the number."

"I like that idea. Beeper to beeper in one year, from callboy to nurse."

"Don't talk that way. I love you."

"Skip, do you know what you just said? You, always so careful with those words."

"I do love you."

"Really? That makes a difference."

"You've done more for me than anyone in my life."

"I'm glad I could, honey, but remember, along with the best times in my life, you've given me some of the worst."

"I want to make up for it. Roger, I'll do anything you want. I'll even be loyal to you. I want the last part of your life to be the best part."

"By 'loyal' you mean 'faithful,' and that's an idea I cannot take seriously. I would not want it even if it were possible."

"Roger, honey, I want to be there when you die."

"I'm sure you will. because you're likely to be the immediate cause of death. But isn't this whole thing a career you're dreamed up while you're between jobs and lovers? It's understood, I'm sure, I'd support you, which I would do, and lay on frequent trips and treats. So you'll transform yourself into loving wife or, more reasonably, son, and me an invalid to be looked after for the duration. If the duration is not unreasonably long."

"Yes, but I care about you, and I do want to look after you."

"Frankly, I'm not sure you'd be very good at looking after anyone. You're a distinctive and beautiful person. You're also a brave little guy, but you don't know much about how the world works. My secretary, Sarah, knows ten times as much. Ten times as much as either of us."

"I could learn."

"In spite of all the problems, I admit I'd like to think of you as a son or wife or something and take care of you and try to make you happy. I need such a person, but not because I need to be taken care of. Your qualification is very simple. For whatever reason—and I don't know the reason—you arouse feelings in me of a kind that no one else does—except Grant, and he's taken himself out of my life."

"Isn't that what I've been saying? What should we do for our anniversary August 17?"

"I know the answer. A road company of *Phantom of the Opera* is coming to town on August 6 and we should see *Phantom* again. Remember when we saw it in New York and, in the middle of the first act, you decided it was our story: A hideously scarred older man promotes the career of a beautiful young singer and is rewarded with her love. Until he removes his mask, and she screams and faints."

"And after, you waved your hands like Dracula and said: 'Sing for me, Christine!' And we giggled all the way back to the Pierre. *Phantom*'s perfect."

"There's just one thing, Skip," I said. "If I'm going to give up dream boys and we're going to have this very close relationship, we'll have to have sex."

"How often?"

"Once a week."

"What day?"

"How about Friday?"

"Make it Monday. Monday's a rotten day anyway."

"You little prick, you think you can say anything to me!"

"Actually, I haven't had sex with anyone since you started seeing me again in April. That's about three months, Roger."

"I don't believe it! Why?"

"Out of respect for you."

"But, Skip, I've never asked such a thing. We're not lovers, never have been. And even if–I'd expect you to be active at the gym or wherever. I just wouldn't ask about it and it wouldn't bother me."

"It's probably good for me. Sex ruled my life. Now, thank God, I have you in my life."

* * *

Skip became very affectionate and attentive, calling, for instance, several times a day, ending with a silly "tuck-in" call. Not so silly after all, as Roger, now 67 years old, was picking up infirmities, and glad for sympathy from anyone. The most troublesome of the infirmities was spinal stenosis, an arthritic narrowing of the spine at lumbar levels four and five which pinched nerves in my right leg and set two blocks as the upper limit on his walking.

I told Julia Child about this problem at a dinner party Rebecca gave for all her food friends, which included most of the chefs and restaurant critics in Boston. Julia said: "I have it too; it's very aging, don't you think?" I laughed: "Aging? Julia, I'm aged." She, I knew, was eighty.

"I like your little escort." Skip had come with me and distinguished himself in a game played at dinner. Everyone was to say what he or she would order as a last meal, supposing every food and wine on earth to be available. The cuisine cognoscenti made it a contest of esoteric knowledge, and their truffles and trifles and vintages went beyond Skip's experience–and mine. But when Skip's turn came he said, "I'd have chocolate cake with chocolate icing and a quart of cold milk," and the company collapsed. Skip enjoyed the party and created one of his funniest routines with Julia.

"I like your little escort. More wine, Rebecca! Do you suppose he could escort me occasionally? More wine, Rebecca!" All in the unique Julia Child voice, just slightly exaggerated.

Skip and I had been talking all July and early August about a trip to Morocco, but now it was jeopardized by the half-crippled right leg. Al and I had gone to Morocco in February of 1965, and I remembered it as the best trip we ever made.

"We landed in Tangiers and by the time we had unpacked there was a line of boys at the hotel gate offering their services to us. We adopted one especially sweet-looking boy and he guided us all over Morocco. Fez, Tiznit, Taroudant, Marrakech. It amazes me that I can still remember the names after something like twenty years. Then we drove over the Atlas mountains and I still remember coming around a curve to one of the greatest sights of my lifetime. The mountains fell away precipitately, without foothills, to the blazing Sahara."

Skip caught the special excitement with which I told my "Tales of the Casbah," and was wild to go, but after watching me limp around for several weeks he made a decision: "We're not going to Morocco."

"Could I possibly have a cheap car since we're not going to Morocco?" Not quite Skip's next line but it followed hard upon. "It's my dream to have a Geo Tracker and they only cost $12,000."

"A Geo Cracker? I never heard of it."

"Tracker, you weenie, not Cracker. It's a really cool car. Small, somewhere between a jeep and a truck. It's exactly right for me."

So Skip and I drove to the nearest dealer in Geo Trackers (or Crackers). Skip talked on the phone with his brother to find out how to get the best prices.

"The first thing I'll do is ask to see the invoice. Then I'll tell him we'll be paying cash. His eyes will go out on stalks. I think I'll start at eleven-five and go to twelve. There's no way he's going to let us out of the store without making a deal if he has $12,000 cash."

Both Skip and I had put on suits and ties in order to intimidate the salesman. He proved to be a careless young man who came to work in his shirtsleeves and impertinently addressed the professor without title. And so it was Skip and Roger who felt intimidated.

We went out to the lot and looked at a glistening black Geo Tracker (or Cracker) with power steering, power brakes, and AM-FM stereo. Skip squandered some bargaining power when he sighed: "It's my dream." The price on the sticker was a terrifying $15,237.09.

Seated at a table ready to drive a hard bargain, Skip said: "We're paying cash. What can you do for us on the price?" I took out my checkbook and held a Mont Blanc pen poised for writing.

"We actually prefer time payments. The profit to the dealer is larger that way. There's very little markup on an inexpensive car like this, but I'm authorized to come down $1,000." That would be $14,237, not the $12,000 Skip had told me it would cost, and I had already expressed shock on hearing insurance the first year would be $2,000.

"That's too high. May we see the invoice, please?"

"Sure, I'll get it from the office."

I whispered: "Skip, what exactly is an invoice?"

"I don't know. I thought you would know."

"Here's the invoice. As you can see the cost to us is $13,711, so if we sell the car at $14,237, our profit is dick!" I wished there were some even numbers and round figures in the automobile business.

"How much did you expect paying?"

"A top of $12,000."

"As you can see, that's out. It'd cost us almost two grand."

Skip stole a look at me to see if I was about to walk out. But no, I'd got caught up in the game. "Could you shave off the $237.00 and let us have it for an even $14,000? You'd still be making a profit of almost $300.00."

"*I* certainly couldn't. We can talk to the boss and see what he says."

In a large private office a splendid-looking gentleman rose to shake hands with Skip and me and was introduced to us as Mr. Cronkite. "All right Skip and Roger, we're all busy men here, so let's not waste anyone's time. The absolute minimum price on this little car is $14,111."

"What about extras? Skip, does this car have everything on it that you want?"

"Power steering and brakes, radio and cassette."

"Cassette player's another $300."

A new car without a cassette player would be for Skip, singer and composer, like no car at all. His dream was a music box on wheels.

"You'll also need a Lo-Jack antitheft device. Reduces your insurance 30 percent and pays for itself in three years." I was not up to doing percentages just now, but guessed that the final cost would be around $18,000, not the $12,000 of Skip's estimate. This would empty my checking account. I turned to look at Skip.

The determined wheeler-dealer was gone, replaced by a boy so close to his dream but watching it evaporate. A boy, I thought, brave and cheerful and sweet-natured through much adversity. Skip's eyes glistened; his tiny facial tic was fluttering.

I said: "Okay, fine, we'll take it with all the extras, all the good stuff."

Skip's misted eyes looked into mine. "I can't believe you're doing this for me."

"It's about time someone did something for you."

* * *

In mid-August Skip's interest in the little drama he had fashioned began to wane. Not at all precipitately and not in any way that hurt me. He got a job at a mental health center, taking care of schizophrenic patients ("clients," he corrected me) in a closed ward. He was extremely good at it, because of his kind heart, vitality, and strong stomach. The hours were rough and the pay was low, but he got a health plan and a pension plan and was interested in the work.

Skip also moved. Not to Cambridge (too expensive) but Southie (South Boston). He got his own studio apartment, and I helped him finance a modest furnishing—everything distinctive because Skip made the choices. Skip also gave up the life of abstinence and got involved once again with people his own age. I thought I might eventually feel neglected.

But just in the nick of time Grant called. What to do?

Jack told me: "You really need two boys. At any given time, one of them's going to be treating you like shit."

* * *

Grant suggested dinner at our favorite place, Legal Sea Food.

"I haven't gone anywhere. I just needed some space. How come you don't ask me if we can go back to the way we were? That seems a conspicuous omission."

"Grant, I haven't seen you in over a month. I felt totally dismissed. You say you haven't gone anywhere, but you only turned heterosexual and moved out of town."

"I never dismissed you, and I know I'm not heterosexual. A month isn't a long time. I guess you never understood I'm a very constant person."

When the two of us were walking back to my apartment, my right leg went into a kind of spasm and I had trouble walking.

"Put your arm around my neck and lean on me."

"Are you sure? There are people around."

"I don't care; if anyone doesn't like it I'll smash them. We can hold hands if you want to."

"That's some change. You asked why I don't ask to go back to the way we were. That's a hard question. I wish I could escape it but you've always been absolutely straight, and I owe you a straight answer. In crude terms the answer is that I've gone back to Skip. But that is too crude. Skip and I never did have sex together and don't now. I do love him and I think he even loves me. I won't give him up. I also can't give you up. To ask me to choose would be like asking a man to choose between two sons."

"That won't be necessary," and Grant added: "Let's go back and fool around."

"My right leg is killing me."

"We won't need your right leg."

* * *

In the late summer of 1992, Grant had an idea for a business venture but no venture capital. He did not ask me for anything–ever. Not a penny, but in the next four months Grant accepted something like sixty thousand dollars. I gave it out of a desperate need for

Grant to experience success and to experience it soon, before the illness came that inevitably must. I did not think about gratitude but I must, of course, have hoped to gain something.

I knew nothing about business, but I was not optimistic about Grant's project. It was to sell shower curtains printed with Italian Renaissance masterpieces, one masterpiece to a curtain. It sounded a little less arbitrary as you added particulars. The curtains would not be made of plastic but of a high-quality cotton that looked almost like linen. The pictures were all in the common domain and so there would be no major copyright costs. Reproductions would be achromatic, black-grays-white, and so cheaper than color, but also very unlike the originals. Grant figured he could sell them for $30 or even a bit less.

But it sounded like a blind man prospecting for gold. What made Grant think people would be attracted to shower curtains with bad prints of centuries-old paintings? On this one point Grant had a little privileged information. He was friendly with two wealthy men, Beacon Street residents, who owned a business called Graphiques de Qualité. Graphiques sold fine reproductions of Old Masters to businesses all over the United States and Europe. At dinner with these gentlemen he read the names of the three most popular pictures on which there was a worldwide consensus: Botticelli's *Venus*, *God Creating Adam* from Michelangelo's Sistine Chapel, and Flandrin's *Jeune Homme Nue*. All the pictures happen to be Renaissance creations (more or less) and that fact gave rise in Grant's uncritical mind to the generalization that people today are drawn to something, actually nonexistent, that he called "the Renaissance look."

To add substance to the hunch, Grant, in conversation with Jack and me, asked questions like: "What do you think of when I say 'Renaissance'?" Most of the answers were noncorroborative: "the *Mona Lisa* or "those intricate detailed drawings by da Vinci of engines of war and human anatomy." There was nonetheless some abstract support in their conversations. Jack and I, both being culture-preeners, used Grant's question as an invitation to make creative and esoteric suggestions of our own. Why not Giotto's this or Mantegna's that or Donatello's whatever?

Grant pretended to entertain each suggestion seriously, and incidentally gave the impression that he knew the works referred to, but in his mind he was loyal to the original three. This was actually just because he himself belonged to the worldwide population that could identify the three, however distorted, on whatever material, and even dripping wet.

Grant gave Jack and me a second chance to make his project momentous by simply posing another question that opened opportunities to show off. What should the name of his company be? Grant had thought "ICON." "What does 'icon' mean to you?" An opening for Roger, the student of signs and symbols.

"Technically, an 'icon' is a sign that suggests its sense in some way. In any way at all. Onomatopoeic words that imitate sounds, like 'cock-a-doodle-doo' for the call of the rooster, are icons of a sort. You may think 'cock-a-doodle-doo' very unlike the rooster's call, but if I tell you that in another language it is 'kiki-ri-ki' and in still another 'coque-li-co,' you may notice all use multiple syllables and so are in segments, as is the call. Most syllables start with consonants that are 'plosives,' which means sudden, not gradual, onsets of sounds, as is the way of the rooster's segments. No language uses anything like 'meow' for the rooster."

Jack and Grant rolled their eyes at what was beginning to sound like a lecture, and not a newly minted lecture at that. But my professional deformation kept me from noticing and I steamrolled on.

"An icon can also suggest its sense by imitating the shape of a referent or miming some action associated with it. Most of the signs of the American Sign Language and probably all signed languages are icons in this sense." And I did my exaggerated versions of the two, the only two, I could always remember. With thumbs interlocked and palms inward, I fanned my hands up and down: BUTTERFLY. With the left hand shaped as a cylinder, I used my right as if screwing on a lid: JAR.

Since Grant and Jack had not enrolled in this course for credit, they interrupted. "It's not really that sense of 'icon' I had in mind," said Grant. "Isn't an icon also a sacred object, like a religious picture?"

"Exactly," Jack chimed in. "You must remember the Rublov icons in Russia, Roger, the small religious paintings put up in households, often with a single candle. The Boston Museum has several hundred of them. In this sense the Renaissance paintings could be considered icons. But, as a name for your business, I wouldn't spell it in the usual way with a 'c.' IKON with a 'k' is much more striking, I think, and in a way appropriate. With a 'k' the word looks like Greek and echoes Greece, the mother of the Renaissance."

Grant rolled his eyes and smiled at me. "You don't think that's just a teensy bit esoteric? You gentlemen have just sold me on ICON. I've got the name, then, but I'm not having a logo designed or stationery. Lots of businesses do it even before the product and then fail. First comes the product. Then the failure. Just kidding."

Now I had to abandon my theory that Grant had no follow-through. Grant became an engine of infinite energy. Even the side effects of the drugs he took for Beth Israel's AIDS experiment did not slow him. He tracked down copyrights for particular reproductions—and this could mean writing a dozen letters for a single picture. Sometimes there was a user fee, and if this were not small, Grant's budget demanded that he give up that reproduction. All the while he was learning the steps in the production process, buying fabric, printing, packaging, finding out who did these things, for how much money, and where they were. He traveled to small towns in New England and Pennsylvania, inspecting equipment and talking terms. This was accomplished in Grant's own heroic style on little money and with maximal physical punishment— driving trucks all night, flying puddle jumpers, swinging on ropes, and shooting rapids. Then he decided he had to move again, now to New York City.

Grant's goal was to have prototypes of the three curtains for the textile design show in New York, October 12-15, so he could take orders and line up salespeople to represent ICON. He needed a small office in the city, a telephone, and a fax machine. Amanda lived in New York in the house she got out of her divorce settlement; she could give Grant a bedroom and was willing to work full-time as office help on spec.

I was unhappy about the all too conjugal arrangement between Grant and Amanda. I said it sounded as if they were bound to become lovers, and Grant laughed. "I taught Amanda scuba diving in Hawaii six years ago." The implication, I presumed, was that if Grant had been disposed to become a lover to Amanda he would have done so then and been done with it.

I could stand the workweeks, as I imagined them, because I saw Grant on weekends. For just four weeks. And then only on Sundays. Mondays Grant had to go to Beth Israel for poking and prodding.

I insisted Grant stay at the Ritz and have good meals and a massage and a little luxury as a change from the life that he depicted as unremitting toil: New York. "It takes everything I've got to hold this business together. All I do is work and sleep. I work every evening, all evening. Last week I even forgot to masturbate." I believed everything as long as Grant was there, with his clear-eyed gaze, saying it. Jack didn't believe any of it, he would tell me on the phone, but in Grant's company, he rolled over like a puppy.

I introduced Grant to Kenny, the Ritz doorman: "I'd like you to meet my son," and my tone said: "In whom I am well pleased." Long after Grant was gone, Kenny would ask: "Is your son here with you? How is he? Tell him I said hello."

"I don't need to stay at the Ritz; I can sleep anywhere."

"I like you to have that little extra comfort."

"I could put the money to much better use."

"This money is not otherwise available to you."

One weekend Grant was frantic. If he were to have an initial run of shower curtains in time for Christmas, it would have to be ordered at once. A minimal run would cost $10,000. He could see no way to do it.

A knock on the door and a delivery of white roses for Grant Flag. From Amanda. The card read: "Don't worry. Things will work out."

"That's really sweet," said Grant. "You notice there's one yellow rose. In the language of flowers this means 'Not in love, but in friendship.'"

Roger, not familiar with the language of flowers, said: "Hmmm." In fact, Amanda was right, and things did work out. On Sunday Roger sat down and wrote a check for $10,000, payable to ICON.

* * *

Another weekend there was a blizzard, and Jack waited with me for Grant, who was long overdue. Jack had grown increasingly disaffected with Grant, as much out of his own frustrated passion as anything to do with Grant. In spite of this, Jack felt sorry to see me today hurting so at Grant's neglect.

Finally the phone rang. "Yo, it's me. I jus' called La Guardia."
Was there a slight slur in Grant's speech? "They say the airport is
closed because of the storm. I fear I can't get there t'night."

"Why didn't you leave earlier?"

"Because, because . . . I couldn't get my work finished in the
office."

The instant I hung up Jack leaped on the phone. "Hello, Trump
Shuttle, are flights from New York cancelled? No? Is La Guardia
closed down? I thought not. Thank you." Rubbing his hands and
chortling: "We've got him this time. Call him back, the lying bastard."

"Grant, Logan says La Guardia is not closed and all flights are
on time. You can still make the six o'clock."

"Weally? I mean, really? I got a recorded message. Obviously
shupersheded." All in a swashbuckling tone, somewhat undercut
by the slur.

About 7:30 Grant called from the Ritz, very happy: *"J'arrive!
J'arrive!"* I liked to hear Grant switch into his awful French. It
always meant he was carefree again, back in the time before the
lead ceiling closed over him. And probably he was drunk.

"Stay there, Grant, I'll be right over."

"I'm going upstairs for a m–massage."

"Okay, I'll see you in the room."

Jack, grimly judgmental, and Roger sat in the hallway outside
room 536 waiting for Grant. The big oaf came looping down the
hall, let them into his room, and collapsed giggling on the bed. He
patted the space beside him and motioned me over.

"I ask him why he wa' spending so much time on my ass and
aroun' my crotch. I *certainly* hope you're not gay–a masseur at the
Ritz!"

Jack frowned. "What have you taken?"

"Special K. No, K. It's a tranquilizer. An animal tranquilizer. For
big animal, like me, 'n horshes 'n cows. No, not cows. Bulls." He
let his cock flop out of his boxer shorts and giggled uncontrollably.
Joined by Roger.

But not Jack. "It's the latest street drug. Very strong. No one
knows how it acts on humans. Probably it inhibits the frontal cortex
and activates the limbic system."

"I was feeling depressed this morning and a friend gave me this." He held up a cube of sugar, turned brown. "I think we all s'do K together on the bed. It'll be a male bonding experience. Nothing queer about that."

Roger, ever game, reached for the cube.

"You don't eat it! You shmell it. Sniff it. That's it. Three times. Now, jus' wait. Here, Jack."

"Not me."

"Why? Don't be so prim."

"I don't know anything about that stuff."

Grant turned a bemused smile on me, held it, and then very slowly raised one supercilious eyebrow. Higher and higher it went; impossibly high. The entire side of his face slid up after the eyebrow like geological strata in an earthquake. Then everything in the room began to roll toward a vortex that contained me and Grant. This was the professor's only experience of a consciousness-altering drug, and I was glad it only lasted four minutes.

Later, as we were leaving, Jack slipped me the sugar cube. "Don't let him have it back. He could kill himself."

At home alone, undressing for bed, I heard my bell ring and then a violent hammering on his door.

"Give it to me!" Grant's shoulders filled the doorway. Behind him Jack gave a helpless shrug. There was a Boston Coach waiting, and Jack would not hear of my getting all dressed just to drop Grant at the Ritz. Jack would be glad to do it.

Back in room 536, Grant dropped on the bed like a felled tree. Jack tried to pull off his boots but could not, so he just opened his shirt and loosened his pants. Then, like Hamlet coming upon Claudius at prayer, Jack thought: "Now might I do it pat." Grant would be likely to go along, out of good nature and simple animal sensuality. But something deterred Jack. Certainly not loyalty to me, or decency. Probably just cowardice. And he planted a kiss on the cowboy's brow.

The weekend of the design show, October 20-21, the Met was doing *Das Rheingold* at a Saturday matinee, and I decided to go. I was not listening to music these days and, in fact, had pretty much stopped when Albert died. At the funeral, driving out to the cemetery, something incredibly corny had happened. I clicked on the radio, which was always set at WCRB, and out came "Addio, fiorito asil," Pinkerton's farewell to Butterfly, sung by Carlo Bergonzi. I started crying, then sobbing convulsively, almost choking.

All very operatic, not only Puccini but Puccini's biggest tearjerker, *Madama Butterfly*. For more than a year, overreaction was the problem with music. Not just Puccini but any music, even movie music, even Bach, was too much for me. It acted as an amplifier of grief, whether or not it was music to grieve by, and I could not take it except at those times, when, in private, face buried in Albert's pillow, I just let go and howled.

When I began to get better in 1991, the problem with music reversed; overreaction was replaced by underreaction. Listening to *Parsifal* in the spring of 1990, I felt nothing at all. Whatever turned off the grief, whatever brain chemical stopped sending sorrow, also stopped decoding the meanings in music.

And so Roger, who had listened to music most of his life, stopped. He also stopped having feelings on the deep level that Albert tapped (though not, we know, in the shallows of jealousy, desire, anger, and resentment). Every now and again Roger would notice the triviality of his emotional life. He seemed to have moved from tragedy to hassles and would sometimes hunger for transcendence. It was just this hunger for transcendence that put him in the mood for *Das Rheingold* in October of 1992.

"I'm coming to New York this weekend, Grant."

"You are?"

"To see *Rheingold* at the Saturday matinee."

"Of course, the Met is doing Wagner; you're a Wagner fan, so you're coming to town."

"I'm coming Friday afternoon and leaving early Sunday. If you have any time, I'd very much like to see you."

"You should have told me. This is the weekend of the show, and we're rushing around trying to put the exhibit together. Turns out you have to rent a space and register in advance. I didn't know, and the spaces are all taken. Today I walked all over the hall and found a little corner that isn't rentable. So I put on my blue suit and made a forlorn pitch to the committee—let me use the space, help a young guy get started."

"I'm sure they found you irresistible."

"Naturally. Now we have to hang the curtains and think up some way to make an attractive booth."

"Who's 'we'?"

"Amanda and I, of course. She's been just great."

"I'd like to meet her. How about Friday night dinner? With Amanda."

"Some old friends of mine from Michigan are in town and we're supposed to see them, but I don't think we're going to make it; there's just too much to do with the booth."

"Well, how about Saturday?"

"Saturday, we said we'd watch the World Cup at some friends' house, but I don't think we'll make that either."

"I thought you didn't have a social life in New York."

"Ordinarily I don't, but you had to pick the worst weekend of the year."

"Okay. Call me at the hotel Saturday and let me know how the curtains go over. I'm really anxious to know." I had not seen the curtains, but I did not think they were likely to go over well. One of my reasons for coming to New York this weekend was, as they say, to "be there" for Grant if the curtains flopped. To commiserate, to help defend his self-esteem and figure out what next.

Grant called just before noon. "Roger, it's fantastic! We're the talk of the show! I've been interviewed by two magazines! I've written orders for Macy's and Barney's! And for a buyer in Hong Kong! Small, but they're orders. Roger, we're not just going to Morocco; we're going on safari!"

In my mind I thanked God, that Grant should have this success, this confirmation of his talents. And have it now while he still felt completely well.

I had a big success once. With my 1965 *Social Psychology*. The experience was so exhilarating that, while it lasted, it seemed to compensate for all the rotten luck in life, even being queer. I could hear that now in Grant's voice. Shower curtains could do it as well as books. To be chosen! To be right! To be acclaimed! Fifteen minutes of fame!

"It's wonderful, Grant. When can I come down to see the booth?"

"Come at three; it'll be less busy. They won't let you in without a
badge; just tell them to come and get me at ICON's display. Everyone knows where it is."

The show was a shock to me. Acres and acres of junk. Directly
opposite ICON stood a very large display of things made of satin
with pleats and frills; what were they, anyway—pillows or futons?
Or just poufs? "Nice stuff," I said to the presiding salesman.

In this assemblage, Grant, taller than anyone else and, in his dark
blue suit and rep tie with the purple and green stripes, more elegant,
looked like a prince come for a visit. The shower curtains looked
damn good. They possessed the classy look Grant had sweated for
and made everything else look shoddy. Once I saw the curtains I
knew they would sell. I wanted one myself. I said to Grant:

"How did you know?"

"I think it's called 'vision.' "

"Either that or you're terrifically lucky. Some people try to hit it
right all their lives. You're going to be a rich man. Then it will be
'Good-bye Roger.' " I was kidding.

"The Botticelli and Michelangelo are both immensely popular
but the nude young man is not. The buyers all say the same thing,
even use the same word: 'Too risqué.' " I wondered at the semantic
imprecision. The beauty of the picture lay in the naturalness, its
unstudied character. It was at the furthest extreme from risqué,
which had a Folies Bérgère ring to it.

I got a quick look at Amanda; something small and middle-aged
and sweet and timorous ran off as I arrived. Grant introduced us, but
it was a hurried, ill-formed encounter, and Grant told me afterward
Amanda asked who the distinguished-looking old man had been.
One could hardly say that we had met. But it was as close as we
would ever come.

The show was closing for the day. Grant packed up the ICON
display. I watched and tried to feel included, standing first on one
foot and then the other, a stage-door johnny. Grant seemed not to
feel any responsibility for me, and I thought he might just walk off
without a word.

"It's pretty clear, I guess, you don't have any time tonight."

"I'll call you later. I'm tired out. What I need now is a shower
and something to eat."

I went back to the hotel. I was dead certain there would be no call. I called a number listed in *The Advocate*: "Two Israeli hunks; just watch or join in." I needed the option, and whichever I chose would serve the purpose, which was to shit on Grant Flag. In the event, I thought I was choosing to join in. But since I could feel no excitement whatever, watching was what it came to, and I was very glad when the two hunks came and went. Knowing the outcomes beforehand, but perhaps wishing to be certain Grant was rotten enough to be terminated forever, I called Amanda's. No answer. "We" had decided to watch the World Cup after all.

The first shuttle in the morning was at six, and I stayed up waiting for it. I wanted out of New York as soon as possible. When Grant should finally bethink himself of Roger, Roger wanted not to be there.

Home at last, pale, unshaven, and feeling sick, I pressed the button to play my messages.

"Roger, what happened? I went to the hotel first thing this morning, thinking we could have a good breakfast together. They told me you already checked out. Why did you leave so early? Please call me when you get this message."

Not today. Not bloody goddamned today. And not ever–if God will give me the strength.

* * *

Thanksgiving night I had a heart attack. Several times that week just before going to sleep I had noticed a fluttering in my chest; it was not painful, but it was something new. I mentioned it to Jack.

"Where exactly do you feel it?"

"Here" (rubbing the center of my chest).

"That's definitely not a heart attack. Cardiac patients never actually touch their chest; they just point." Jack was always so certain and such an asshole about psychosomatic illness. I would never let him forget this false diagnosis.

"You're having a panic reaction. Everything conspires to create it at this time. Your mother died of a coronary. We're approaching the anniversary of Albert's death. And you're struggling to detach yourself from Grant. In effect, it's a time of abandonment and loss of all your strongest object-attachments. How could you not have panic?"

After it was all over, I teased Jack but, in fact, thought him not entirely wrong, at least with respect to the timing of the attack. The timing seemed especially appropriate when Amanda had a heart attack two weeks later. It confirmed my view that Grant was toxic to the people who loved him.

The attack was mild, nothing like the agonies my mother had suffered. It was just that the sensations did not go away and were intensifying, so I called Harvard Health's number and an ambulance whisked me over to Massachusetts General Hospital. They gave me nitroglycerine, which stopped the sensations, and I got up, ready to go.

"You'll have to stay here—at least tonight."

"Oh no you don't. I feel all right and I'm going home if I have to walk. I'll come back for tests." To Roger, who could not stand to have his obsessive routines disturbed, hospitals were like Dachau.

"If you leave, it'll be against doctor's orders."

"So be it."

"You're on the brink of a major attack, but it's temporarily forestalled. If you leave, you could drop dead."

I was not sure that this prospect was worse than life without Grant. However, Jack got a psychiatrist friend in to say my judgment was impaired. So in due course, it transpired that I must have a coronary bypass operation. I could not be put on the operating room schedule for ten days, but Jack used his influence at the hospital to get me a VIP suite in Phillips Brooks House. For ten days I entertained friends and students and received flowers and fruit. It was not terribly different from the Ritz.

The only way in which the operation held any interest for me was as a test of Grant's feeling. Would he realize how much he needed me? Would he fly to my bedside? Not right away, he didn't. Grant told Jack he had to stay in New York to be near Amanda; she had no one else. But then, Amanda's heart attack turned out not to require surgery; it could be treated with medication. And the very next Monday (when Grant had to check in with Beth Israel anyway) he went straight to see me at Mass General.

Grant burst into the room in his winter greatcoat, a hero from a romantic novel. Heathcliff, in fact, a scowl on his brow and mud from the moors on his boots. He swooped down on me, kissing me on the cheek. I appreciated the gesture, because one of my graduate students was there, a gay man, and I was proud to have him see the almost conjugal move.

Alone, the two men talked, together for the first time since New York. Grant was full of excitement; he had thousands of dollars in orders and was working all the time mailing them off, but there was still a significant test ahead: Most of the orders were not "cash on delivery" but were payable in sixty days, and there was really no way to compel payment.

Buyers could place orders, small ones, for anything that appealed to them, and if some things did not sell, they would return the product and just not pay. All Grant had demonstrated at this point was the ability to predict the taste of buyers. The more significant test, just ahead at Christmas, was sales—which would be reflected in payment of the first orders and placement of new ones.

It usually took five years for a new company to show substantial profits, Grant said. And three shower curtains did not make a business. He needed a full line of ICON products, starting with bathroom accessories. He had a lot of ideas but could not find time to design them. He had needed to explain all this to Amanda already, because, as she typed up invoices for thousands of dollars, day after day, she came to think she should be paid something.

"I paid $500 a week but have to stop because everything has to be ploughed back into the business." I blinked, registering the fact that it was my dollars that had been used to pay my rival.

"It's tremendously exciting and I'm very optimistic." Then, taking my hand: "I couldn't have done it without you." I blinked again, and Grant said, "And one or two other people who believed in me."

"Grant, no one comes into this room without knocking. The bathroom door can be locked. I'm going to be cracked open like a lobster on Monday, and God only knows when I'll feel whole again. I want you to come into the bathroom with me and let me make love to you."

Grant chuckled: "Oh no you don't, nothing gross."

"Gross? It wouldn't be gross; it would be the only thing in this antiseptic death house that isn't gross. It would take the curse off the place. It would do what desire and fucking do in Orwell's *1984*, mess up all the inhuman efficiency."

"Here we go again. This time you're not even being persuasive. I've got to get back to New York." And he left.

I hobbled into the bathroom alone. Gross; he thought it would be gross to have sex here. Because we would have had to lie on the floor? Because we would have shared the space with a toilet? I thought my love could only make any place holy. But that was my love. What would Grant's love have been?

I looked in the mirror. It was a mirror lit by fluorescent tubes, a light that took no prisoners. An old man's face. Unrecognizably ugly and evil. All tucks and puckers and slack lines and squinty red eyes. Was this the face Grant saw inviting him to make love in the toilet?

I groaned: "Poor Grant! What have you suffered?" And then I thought: Why have you suffered it? I never could have. It can only have been for the money. It must have taken a strong stomach and a strong purpose. I think you have a plan, Grant. A plan for the rest of your life. A desperate plan, because you know the rest of your life may not be long. I have played my part and you are just about through with me. If the business succeeds, you will be able to get out of New York, taking your phone number and fax machine, and live somewhere, the way you want to live, outdoors all year.

* * *

Jack and Edwige and Skip all came to look in on me while I was in Recovery. Skip later told me I looked beautiful in coma, and he tied to my bed a carved wooden heart, painted red, reading: "Keep your chin up; I love you." Edwige cried. Jack took over as closest relative. He called Marian, Joan, and my family, and my friends and colleagues called Jack for medical bulletins.

Jack was never fond of long talks on the telephone and far too busy anyhow. He made an exception with Grant. Grant called often, and Jack gave him medical details. Essentially what Grant was asking, however, was: "Should I come?" shading off into "Do I have to come?" Jack cooperated with Grant's clear wish to be spared. "I don't think it's necessary. There's not really anything you could do that we're not doing, and he feels too rotten most of the time to carry on a conversation. No, he has not asked for you." This was a great unkindness to me, and Jack knew it but could not resist interposing himself between the two men.

In my mind I did nothing but call for Grant. It was true that I did not ask for him. My life-threatening illness was a test, and its value as such would be destroyed if I begged to see Grant. It was a test bound to have a sad outcome for me, but Jack could perhaps have fudged the results a bit by urging Grant to come and not telling me. He chose instead to let me discover how little Grant cared about me.

Back before the heart attack, Grant and I had spoken of getting together at Christmas in New York. Grant thought he would like to see the *Nutcracker* as the New York City Ballet did it. When the hospital let me go home in mid-December, I thought I would be strong enough for the Christmas Eve performance, and I even had the tickets, bought a month ago on "spec"–which here means speculation as to how things might later be going between Grant and me. As things were going in December, we were talking quite often on the telephone, but I was too tender, not in the incision–that had healed–to raise the subject of Christmas and risk a rebuff. Clearly the *Nutcracker* had been forgotten, and I could not any longer ask Grant to do anything.

Skip wanted to return to the Pierre for Christmas and the idea appealed also to me, but for a week or so I held back from a commitment, especially a Christmas Eve commitment, in case Grant should take it into his head to spend that time with me. Skip saw clearly what I was feeling and forgave it, but it rather spoiled things for him.

Grant did phone. "I'm going to my sister's in Philadelphia for Christmas. My parents'll be there and it's time I came out to all of them. They need to get ready for the shock of AIDS."

Skip and I went to the Pierre for one night and pretended it was as good as the year before, but it wasn't. Grant didn't come out to any of his family because they had been so happy to see him and had made such a fuss over how handsome he was. He could never find an opening. What chiefly disappointed him, though, was that he and his father had not gotten through to one another.

"It would have gone better at home in Montana. We would have gone out to the barn and looked at the horses."

On February 3 the spring term began and I decided it would be best to return to teaching. It was a risky decision. My only course would be a seminar called "Systematic Psychology and Masterpieces of Literature," and the seminar involved only one two-hour meeting a week, so required classroom time would be minimal. The course was always oversubscribed, but admission was only by permission of the instructor, and I always chose just twenty, a magic number that seemed to generate a lively discussion.

There was a required paper each week and reading these, together with my own preparation for each topic, meant at least forty hours work for every two hours on stage. The risk lay in the possibility that I might start the course and then find myself unable to do it at all. The risk to the students and department was great because for this course, my idiosyncratic invention, there was no possible substitute instructor at Harvard or anywhere.

The first three weeks were very dodgy because in the hospital I picked up a skin infection that inflamed and swelled my right leg from foot to knee. It was cellulitis, the same thing Albert had in his right hand in the last week he was at home, and his swollen, acutely painful hand had become the focus of my solicitude. My own infection now seemed to me another step in recapitulating Albert's march to the grave, but Al's painful hand had given me more suffering by far than my own inflamed leg. I had no guilt over the leg.

Such an infection is the devil to cure and only continuous intravenous antibiotics will do it. The first week of term I was hospitalized and, in order to meet my class, given a two-hour pass and a mobile IV hook-up with a bottle and a loop of tubing. The next two weeks I was out of the hospital and a visiting nurse came every morning to check the IV connection and start a new bottle of antibiotics. The nurse warned me that if anything serious went wrong with the IV, a beeper alarm would sound, and then I must rapidly but carefully carry out a set of emergency operations. These I found myself totally incapable of performing. The beeper did go off—several times—and I could only call the nurse and wait to die.

But I didn't die and became familiar enough with the IV to use it as a prop in seminars. It set off my courage in being there at all.

The infection was cured in three weeks; I paid very little attention to it. My mind was either on my course or on Grant. Grant called just twice.

"Yo, Roger, it's me. What's going on? I understand you have cellulitis. That can be bad news. But I hear by the grapevine that you are doing just fine."

What grapevine? I wailed to myself. Is there some grapevine that connects us?

"I'm not sleeping at Amanda's anymore. I don't feel comfortable there, now, so I crash in an apartment over the office. I call it an apartment, but it's not much more than a closet with a futon."

"What went wrong at Amanda's?"

"Oh she has a paying tenant, Mimi Goldberg, and Mimi told Amanda she doesn't like me there all the time. In fact, she's going to move unless things change. Probably Mimi's jealous of Amanda's attachment to me."

Roger to himself: I thought you worked all the time and that the connection with Amanda was just business.

"Also Amanda is a little antsy because a couple of times I've had to yell at her over mistakes she's made. She has no creative ability whatever and no ability to take initiative. Basically I have to tell her everything. And she has the nerve to say she should get a share of the business. Maybe 25 percent. No way is she getting 25 percent of my business."

Roger and Amanda and Grant seemed to constitute some kind of unacknowledged love triangle with the two afflicted lovers only acquainted through the beloved. And just barely acquainted at that. When I told Jack I had called Amanda at home and suggested that we two talk, Jack was delighted. "What a neat thing! It gives the whole mess an added dimension. What did she say?"

"I'm afraid she turned down my invitation. I think she believes she has the more legitimate claim and she hasn't given up hope. She won't risk a conspiracy with me. Grant still commands the chessboard."

* * *

One of the masterpieces assigned to students in my seminar was Shakespeare's *Coriolanus*, and in the spring of 1993 it seemed to me that Caius Marcius Coriolanus was the literary prototype of Grant Flag. I tried making the case to Jack on Friday afternoon.

"Arrogance is one thing; it's a governing trait in both of them. Coriolanus is Rome's greatest general and he wants to become consul, and deserves to become consul, and the Senate chooses him; but this is Rome in the time of the Republic, and so he must also have the voice of the people. But Coriolanus despises the people:

'You common cry of curs, whose breath I hate / As reek o' th' rotten fens.' Not unlike Grant, if you have ever heard him on the subject of the masses."

Jack replied, "He once said 'All my friends are handsome. What is handsome to me?' And you remember his explanation when you suggested that he was Skip's successor."

"Exactly. However, to win the voice of the people, Coriolanus is told he must ask for it kindly. His wonderful answer is: 'Kindly, sir, let me ha't.' And that is humble compared with Grant asking me for the money to start his business. In fact, he never had to ask at all, because I was so besotted he never had to do more than let slip the sums required and the dates."

"That is at least as much your doing as Grant's."

"Integrity. Grant has it and so did Coriolanus. When his mother, Volumnia, and her friends tell him he need only pretend to love the people, he is at first too proud to play the mountebank but finally grits his teeth and says, 'Well, I'll do it.'"

"That's Grant, except that he won't do it. He won't pretend to love either you or Amanda, though he depends on both of you."

"Certainly never has for me, no endearments, no declarations, and precious few gracious words of any kind. So few *and* so precious that I know them all by heart. 'I like you because you make me laugh.' 'I couldn't have done it without you—and a few others who believed in me.' And of course that painfully prophetic 'Thanks for dinner.' Did I ever tell you, Jack, that after the operation Grant said to me: 'I know what you want me to say. You want me to say I love you, and in a way I do, but there's more nurturance in that love than you want'?"

"The boy is no hypocrite."

"One time, when I was testing a theory about the inner life of this Great Sphinx of ours, I said, 'It must often happen to you, must have happened before, that a man—or a woman—falls so much in love as to be willing to do anything for you. This gives you a tremendous power to manipulate, a power you have exercised with both Amanda and me.'"

"That must have rattled his cage."

"Not noticeably; he just let the idiot child prattle on, and I did. 'My theory, Grant, is that you preserve your integrity, and in a sense your manhood, by never encouraging admirers, never saying anything to suggest these feelings are returned. A starvation diet of this kind permits you to think: 'If this weak person wants to do extravagant things out of love for me, that is his business. It's no responsibility of mine!' And I finished, 'Just tell me, Grant, is this accurate or not?' He smiled indulgently and said: 'You and your theories.' "

"But the defining Grant moment comes the end of the third act of *Coriolanus:*

> . . . Despising,
> For you, the city, thus I turn my back:
> There is a world elsewhere." (III, 3, 133-135)

"That's it, Roger, Grant's famous ability to 'walk away from it'–from premed medicine, from Boston, from the 'A' crowd of gay men; and recently he told me, after going on about the success of ICON, 'You know what, Jack, I could turn around and walk away from it at any time.' "

"And I think soon from me. Albert and I saw Christopher Walken play this scene, and I can still feel the desolation he left behind when he made a slow turn and walked off. Whatever happens, I mustn't let Grant play this scene on me."

* * *

The scene was played on Amanda instead. Grant fired her for making mistakes. He said he would pay her for her work as soon as he could. It was Jack who got the story in passing that Amanda's mother had died that same week.

" 'I tell you, Jack, this week has been a bummer for her.' "

"A bummer, Roger! That's what he actually said!"

* * *

My Masterpieces seminar was a kind of inheritance from Albert, who had taught a brilliant course in Shakespeare. He also taught modern drama, but when meeting new people he liked to identify his work as teaching Shakespeare. Most people registered respect but not envy. Only Jack Quilty had made what Albert considered an appropriate response. "What a wonderful way to spend a lifetime!"

That was ten years ago, and the exchange initiated an almost rapturous sympathy between the two.

I inherited Al's teaching copies of all the plays, each one annotated in the margins with a lifetime of information and insight. I also inherited a thousand-volume library of Shakespeare commentary, and as I worked my way into this I discovered that I had lived a lifetime with an immensely learned man who very rarely let his learning show. With Jack Quilty he had shown it, even joyously displayed it, and I realized too late that my own effect may have been to dampen that impulse.

Coriolanus? Coriolanus? Why out of all world literature had I picked this play to ask my class to read? To be sure, I had Grant on my mind and there were the various parallels I had set before Jack and which Jack had found convincing. Was it more than a conceit that came to mind because I was ruminating on Grant?

The rumination could not account for putting the play on the reading list, because the list was made up before the term started, when I did not know that Caius Marcius was a lot like Grant Flag. No, my decision had been made for intelligent, pedagogical reasons. *Coriolanus* was part of a unit on "Group Dynamics in Drama." I knew the play was about one man in opposition to a unanimous majority and the unit included two other plays with that theme: Reginald Rose's *Twelve Angry Men* and Ibsen's *An Enemy of the People.*

There was the incidental fact that Al had written his dissertation on *Coriolanus;* that happenstance was the only reason I even knew the play. But remembering that changed the question from why I had chosen *Coriolanus* to why Albert had chosen it. I realized that Albert never said—probably put off by my ignorance. Al did most of the work and all the writing in Ann Arbor in 1952 when I had gone on ahead to Cambridge. Marian was still in Ann Arbor in the English Department in 1952, and so in 1993 I asked her: "Why do you think Albert chose *Coriolanus?* "

"You have to remember that in English the problem is to find some work that hasn't already been done to death. Especially with Shakespeare."

"I know, but why *Coriolanus?* Why not *Cymbeline* or better, *Pericles?* I read recently a piece by T. S. Eliot in which he argues that *Hamlet* is seriously flawed and tosses off the judgment that

Coriolanus is the most fully realized of Shakespeare's tragedies. I wonder if Al was influenced by that?"

"I don't think so. It's a new idea to me, and Al never said anything about it. It comes back to me now that what he spoke most about was the big scene at the end of the third act. He called it the 'double banishment' scene, which I guess is its standard name in criticism. You probably remember how it goes. The people of Rome and their tribunes banish Coriolanus, and he turns the tables and in effect says: 'You can't banish me; I banish you.' Then he turns his back and walks off saying, 'There is a world elsewhere.' Critics have written about it a lot, mostly about the word 'banish.' It is a performative, a word that performs or accomplishes the act, if the person who uses it has the necessary power or entitlement, and so it is interesting that Coriolanus seizes it from the people."

"I do remember the scene; I remember it well," I said ruefully. Had I gone against Caius Marcius twice in my life? Was Grant the current incarnation of Albert: obdurate, inexpressive, withholding, but principled and impressive?

Albert and I had played the double banishment scene many times, so many that its form was about canonical. As well as comical. Albert's persistent profligacy sent me–how many times?–into a rage, and I would fly off into the night only to return a few hours later. Then would he roguishly say: "I've decided to forgive you." That–when the whole idea had been that I was banishing him from my life. He won every time. Maddening. And when I left for Harvard it was just double banishment again, with me undoing the decisive rupture as fast as I could. No wonder Albert found meaning in *Coriolanus* in 1952 and no wonder I chose it to teach in 1993.

And was I not still playing the game of double banishment–and losing it–with Albert's surrogates, Skip, and now Grant? But it takes more than insight to stop the repetition compulsion.

* * *

With some people, I, like everyone else, have had the experience of receiving much more love than I could return, and have always had it. Why are we so slow to recognize the signs in others? Why, to name a worst case, was I so slow with Grant? Given a certain level of kindness, some affection or the memory of it, the only signs are small failures: forgetting, arriving late, and cutting short. Every one of these small failures is subject to voluntary correction in the interest of a better performance, every one by itself, but the only way to get the whole constellation right is to *feel* as the other hopes you feel. Which is what one cannot manage to do.

"If you've had enough, I'd rather you just told me." So people say when in this spot, and so I had been saying since early July. But the silent defaulter knows better. "Just telling" when passion is high can be explosive; people get hurt. Far wiser to deny any change ("I haven't gone anywhere") and let the realization grow so slowly that when it becomes definite, one has already habituated to the pain.

That is what went on in the winter and spring, and the pace was slow enough that no real explosion occurred. There was, though, one "fast-forward" day when I felt hate–very unusual for me–and Grant felt fear–very unusual for him: Amanda was replaced on the telephone in New York by a male voice that sounded young and virile. "A lover! Grant has had a lover the whole time! Amanda was just a stalking-horse. 'Now could I drink hot blood!'"

"So, Grant Flag, after all your pretensions, it turns out that you're just a faggot schemer. Or confidence man. Now we'll see how much of this you get away with. I suspect you have a police record and I'm going to put a tracer on you." I wondered if I could make a pipe bomb without blowing myself up.

That night Grant called Jack for the first time in three weeks: "Roger is getting evil about all this. Can't you control him?"

On one of Grant's winter weekends in Boston, he and Jack and I made a plan to go together to Naples, Florida. The dates were anchored by Jack's tight schedule. He could leave on Friday, the 23rd of January, be in Naples by early afternoon, and stay until Monday, the 25th. I thought I could start a day earlier, Thursday the 22nd, and stay a day longer, until the 26th. Grant could definitely commit himself for the weekend of the 24th, since the bathroom accessories business was not conducted on Saturday and Sunday, and probably longer, but he would have to let me know. We would all stay at the Ritz in Naples where Grant had a "wonderful time" the year before and I had "one of the best times in my life."

I undertook to integrate the travel arrangements. Boston planes land at Fort Myers, which is an hour's drive from Naples; as the first to arrive, and last to leave, I would rent a car and drive Jack and Grant back and forth, which would be jolly since we would get a convertible, but it did call for advance planning. For three weeks Grant equivocated about his dates, and plans were set and upset until I finally told him, "Why don't you book your flight yourself when you know what you're doing."

I got to Fort Myers on Thursday, picked up the car, and got lost six times before reaching Naples at four. At one gas station I got out of the car, map in tremulous hand, and a fresh young attendant said: "Where ya goin', pop?" Just the boost I needed when getting ready to meet a lover forty years younger than myself.

The beach at Naples reminded me of happy times the previous year, and I spoke of them over the phone to Grant: "Remember the bamboo bridge over the mangrove swamp? Remember the outdoor lunch place where we put our bare feet up? I wish you were already here."

"I'm coming! I'm coming!" Grant said testily. "My plane gets in at two in the afternoon. Can you meet me?"

Need he ask? I actually practiced driving the first part of the route that night so nothing would make me late the next day. On the way back I knew Grant would take the wheel and, without glancing at the map, set new records for speed, accuracy, and Universal Flawlessness.

The three buddies had only one evening together, Saturday, and that was a little disappointing, since no one had thought of making a reservation in the restaurant we preferred. Grant had to catch a noon plane on Sunday. He and I talked very little on the drive but at the airport Grant managed a big hug: "Wonderful time. Shame it had to be so short." He got on a plane to Miami rather than New York in order to see two friends with AIDS, Marius and Tom, while down in their part of the world. I cut short my stay and left with Jack on Monday.

Grant stayed in Miami a full week. I had no message from him and finally had to make a humiliating call to Amanda at home. "Has Grant moved permanently to Florida?"

"No, I think he's coming back on Saturday. Apparently Tom and Marius are feeling well, and they're having a great time."

Several nights that week I lost control and left wild, angry messages on Grant's machine. Once they were there I had no way of erasing them.

"What a slap in the face! You can only fit in one evening with Jack and me and then spend a week with Marius and Tom. I understand that they are sick, but I have been sick all week over this, and by now I should be your first concern as you are mine."

Grant did not deign to telephone but instead sent the following letter dated February 8, 1993:

> Roger,
>
> I am responding to the messages I received on my answering machine over the last two days. I feel sure they are indicative of your true feelings and have left a very sour taste in my mouth. Apparently you don't understand me at all. I cannot be owned, bought, or sold any easier than I can be told how to spend my time. I choose to do the things I do for very good reasons and resent being told by you that I am not at liberty to make such choices. If you don't have the ability to understand this, then it is indeed best that we have nothing to do with each other.
>
> Grant

I would not take Grant's letter as final. I found a valentine with "I love you" distractedly written all over it. Inside I wrote "Just because I can't get along with you and send you nasty messages doesn't mean I don't." And I included a check that I thought Grant was bound to need. It was cashed, and phone calls were resumed. And I demonstrated that I could be a warm good friend instead of an amorous idiot. But still we did not see one another.

On my birthday, April 14, I was unhappy, remembering that a year ago Grant had been so fearless and affectionate as to appear before all my friends with an armful of white flowers: Casablanca lilies, snapdragons, stocks, gladiolus. I called Grant in the New York office.

"Today is my birthday and I claim the privilege of a long talk when you get through work."

"You've jumped the gun. I was planning to call tonight."

We did have a long, warm talk. And next day I sent Grant a wagonload of white flowers.

"Somebody has sent me the most wonderful flowers, and everybody in the office wants to know who." Grant sounded so affectionate that I thought this was a full reconciliation.

On Saturday when Grant was working alone in his office we spoke again. "I'm not feeling great with the new medication, and I hate this city. It doesn't help being on the outs with the people I really care about."

"You're not on the outs with me, honey. I'm just going to keep issuing invitations and won't be offended when you say no. How about Paris in August with Jack and me? He has a conference, and I would go if you went."

"Paris in August? What a terrible idea. Parisians take their holidays in August, and Paris is just a big hot city full of tourists."

"Well, then, how about San Francisco in June again with Marian and Joan? This year they're doing Richard Strauss operas: *Salome*, *Der Rosenkavalier*, and *Capriccio*. Afterwards we could drive up north along the coast."

"San Francisco. Yes, that was a great trip. I'll commit myself to that. Reserving the right to walk out on any of the operas. But don't make the hotel reservation. Let me pick the hotel; I know some small ones less expensive and more interesting than the ones you go to."

"Great. Will you have dinner with me sometime and talk about the future?"

"The future is Florida. New York is a toilet. It's killing me. I've got to live where I can be outdoors."

"That's one of the things I'd like to talk about. Where in Florida?"

"Fort Lauderdale. I went down for two days, and it looks good. I camped out and was just as comfortable as I would have been at the Ritz. My old friend Hank, who loaned me money on his credit cards—at 16 percent interest—is going to relocate with me."

"What about Hank's guest house on the Cape?"

"It's losing money and he wants to sell it. He'll help me with the business."

"When do you think you'll do this?"

"End of the week."

"*This* week? It's already Tuesday. You can't do it that soon."

"No? Hold on, Roger, the woman who owns the building is at the door. Hi, Dot! What are you doing here on Saturday? I'm on the phone. No, don't leave. Roger, I want to talk to Dottie. How about if I call you in a bit?"

Click.

The call did not come in ten minutes. Nor in half an hour. After one hour I knew it would not come that night. After three days it had not come, and I pictured Grant walking offstage: "There is a world elsewhere, and it's Fort Lauderdale." The call would come, of course—eventually—and I decided on what I must do—to save my life.

The call came about four on Friday. Grant was in the highest spirits. "Hello! Who's this?"

"This is Roger."

"Is this Professor Brown of Harvard?"

"Yes, it is."

"What's going on, buddy?"

"Nothing."

"I'm packing! For Fort Lauderdale!"

"Grant, there's someone here. How about calling back *in a bit?*"

"Really? How long?"

"About 45 minutes."

"Call me when you're through."

"No, you call me."

Click.

I took the phone off the hook. I left the phone off the hook for five days and five nights. When I put it back on, Skip called and Jack called and Rebecca called. Grant never called again, and I did not call him again, ever.

But every time my phone rang, I hoped to pick it up and hear Grant's voice:

"Yo, Roger, it's me. What's going on?"

Finally, eleven months later, there came another kind of call. I was home alone at 6:15. Incredibly, it was Amanda: "Roger, I don't think anyone else knows to tell you. Grant Flag is dead. They say he died in his sleep. It was in a New York hotel. He was here representing ICON."

After Amanda called, I started crying and did not stop for a while. I think of him many times every day, but I have not grieved as I would have done if we had not broken off ten months earlier. Three times in those ten months I called his business number in Fort Lauderdale and heard his young male receptionist answer "ICON," and then I hung up. I meant the break to be forever unless, as I hoped, he would relent and call me. I think I expected him to fall ill from one of the opportunistic infections eventually and thought that would effect a reconciliation, but it seems he never did.

Amanda said her understanding was that he could not void his urine the night before and in the morning he was dead. Some kidney disease, she thought, but she did not know and was herself hungry for information. I thought he might have killed himself, since he twice told me he would if he developed full-blown AIDS, because he would never let himself look like those patients got to looking. I believed him, because it was consistent with both his vanity and his control: "I never do anything I don't want to do." Amanda thought it would not have been suicide because she understood he looked as magnificent as ever.

I never made any phone calls or inquiries because nothing circumstantial mattered any more. Jack, however, could not properly grieve in ignorance and did what detective work was possible. Grant had been joined in Florida by Hank, the friend from the Cape with whom he went on a trip when Grant and I first met. Hank had lent Grant money for ICON, and Grant had meant Hank to have ICON when he died, but there was no will and the Montana family was fighting for it.

Hank loved Grant, but I don't think they ever made love. Grant once said to me: "I wonder what Hank thinks about us. He probably thinks if he had a lot of degrees and stuff I'd let *him* lie down with me." Those were really his words. It seems he let me lie down with him.

I got many things wrong. The receptionist boy was not a lover. Grant never had sex with Amanda. Grant probably had infected Tom and Marius many years ago and that explains the weeklong stay in Miami about which he would only say: "I choose to do the things I do for very good reasons." The Marine Corps, some time before Michigan, threw Grant out because they learned he was gay. That explains the only keepsake he ever gave me: a just-for-fun mock dog tag:

FLAG, G.
USMC
SAGITTARIUS
VERSATILE

Chapter 7

Patrick

In the end I may simply have grown weary of repetition. You can only make a given set of moves a certain number of times before they grow stale. Or it may simply be that I was older (69) and less energetic and finally realized that I must settle for something less than my ideal love. Then, too, there is geographic separation; Patrick, living some of the time in Boston and some of the time in Miami and some of the time in Los Angeles while I stay in Boston. Patrick, bless him, credits me with having learned something.

In February of 1995 he said: "I have to congratulate you."

"You mean because I haven't left you any more nasty phone messages? And am willing to let you call from time to time as you feel like it rather than every single day? I can learn after all. I have learned many things in my life."

"Still, I want to congratulate you."

He was right to do so because what I learned with him I might have learned with Albert or with Skippy or with Grant. They all had made it quite clear. Grant had even written it down: "You need to give me more space if we are to continue spending time together."

It was not that Patrick had had more experience in life; Patrick was my youngest—only twenty-four when we met. He may have had the lesson more poignantly in mind because he was just coming out of a marriage in which he had played my hapless part. "I was just like you with her (his beautiful Thai 'ex'). I wanted to control everything she did but you can't control another person."

Patrick gave me lessons in the impossibility of control almost from the start but they did not change me. Indeed, for a long time it looked as if we were headed for another repetition—the worst ever, and the most ludicrous—an old man already in his pajamas at 9 p.m.

213

shouting at a boy far away in Miami that he suspected the boy of infidelity. I may as well confess that I never learned as much as Patrick gave me credit for. I was as jealous as ever and only learned not to make a record of it.

In the winter of 1993, when Grant was still alive but in New York and long since out of communication with me, I called an escort agency that advertised on a national level, and in high-class media, with a brash and desperate inquiry: "Do you ever have anyone truly spectacular?" Clearly I had recovered from my first-night nerves. Without feeling any better than ever about my body I had decided that it did not matter a damn in what was simply an economic exchange.

The voice that answered was not your usual male madam but more like a cultivated dealer in antique books: "As it happens we have right now a young man who can, without exaggeration, be called 'spectacular.' His fee is also spectacular: 300 dollars." Oddly enough I found this reassuring. I had learned that there are no bargains in this business and 300 hundred dollars was quite the largest fee anyone had ever dared to quote me. This was Boston, after all, not Beverly Hills.

The young man who appeared that evening was just twenty-four-years-old and just under six feet tall. He offered no ingratiating smiles and did not waste time with conversation, but stripped down and presented himself to me in a fronto-parallel plane. Behold me! A centerfold come to life in your living room. Think yourself fortunate.

"You are indeed spectacular, Patrick, and have no competition in Boston!"

"Somebody else told me that recently. My penis is kinda' small though."

"But perfect. Didn't anyone ever introduce you to the concept of a pretty penis?" His was cherry red and so stiff it quivered. "You wouldn't want a grey donkey-dong on your body."

"You have the most perfect butt I've ever seen."

"Everyone tells me that, both men and women. It's also always clean. I figure that's the dirtiest part of the body so whenever I go to the bathroom I take a long hot shower afterwards."

Then without specific intent to please, I said just the right thing: "You must be an M.I.T. student, or Harvard. I can tell by the intelligence and seriousness of your face."

"I *am* intelligent and serious but I never even finished high school. I don't believe in schools. They don't teach you what you need to know."

"What do you do besides escorting?"

"I entertain by dancing and stripping in gay clubs all around the country. Right now I'm takin' naked showers at the Ramrod. You could see my show some night if you wanted to. I also travel as an escort; I have an agent. There's a man in L.A. wants me to come out for a day for $1,000 and someone here wants me to spend the weekend at the Hamptons for $500. I don't go nowhere just for the money; I have to like the person."

"It sounds as if you're a world-class escort—my first." Privately I thought that Grant could have been one but he wouldn't have wanted to.

"What kind of men do you meet on calls like this?"

"Men like yourself."

Clearly he had no idea how crushed I would be to hear that there was nothing to distinguish me from the "others."

"Are you straight or are you gay?"

Patrick smiled a little and said as if repeating a diagnosis someone had made: "I guess I'm sexually confused. Until a few weeks ago I was married to a beautiful Thai girl, Mia. I loved her very much; I still love her, but I let her make a trip to New York and she did what I knew she'd do; she fucked other guys. We had terrific fights."

"Physical fights?"

"Definitely. She had a restraining order put on me. Now I'm suing her and she's suing me. Once I heard her tell lies in the courtroom I turned against her and against all women."

"You don't expect to get married again?"

"Never. I know women's wiles and I'll never fall for them again. I can get myself off better than any woman can. And men can give me pleasure just as well. Though I can't stand faggots. Why would they want to act like they do?"

"It's beyond me."

"I spend most of my time alone or else with straight guys like my roommate Mack. Only he's plannin' on getting married. I try to talk him out of it."

"I am so intimidated by your good looks that I don't want to have sex. Not this time. But I would like to see you soon again, Patrick."

"How often do you get lonely?"

"It's more than loneliness. I have strong feelings for you already."

"That's cool. I like you too."

"Can I hug you?"

"Of course."

"Can I kiss you?"

"I don't like kissin', with either men or women. I never did. I'm kinda squeamish about that."

"I hope to see you again in a few days, Patrick. Is $400 enough for this time?"

"Sure."

* * *

Only two days later I called the agency and asked for Patrick.

"I'll have to ask him. He got food poisoning last night and has been sick all day."

Patrick said, "I guess I can make myself available to that particular gentleman."

Looking slightly squeamish he nevertheless stripped down like a good soldier and presented himself before me in evident expectation of a blow job which I was not this time reluctant to undertake, but when he did not climax after a time and the whole thing began to feel like work I said: "Look, Patrick, I can't do it in this mechanical way as if you'd dropped your car off for an oil change. With some people I could but with you I can't. There has to be some feeling, some emotion. I know that sounds crazy for an escort date."

"You can't buy feelin's."

"I know that, but I have some already. The question is whether you have any."

"I feel different than usual or I wouldn't be here."

"So let's relax about getting off and just get to know one another a little better."

"What do you want to know?" (a little belligerently)

What I most wanted to know was why he had not finished high school but I judged that too tricky a subject to open with.

"Why don't you lie down beside me and let me see that beautiful butt as we talk." He obliged but said: "I can't take it in me. It doesn't turn me on and I think it's unsafe. I was happy to lay my head on the pillow his rump created. "What is your dream, or fantasy, for your life?"

"I have more than a dream; I have a plan. Escorting is just temporary. If I'm lucky, very lucky, I'll break into modeling or even acting. That's the dream, I guess, but it's every escort's dream and I know it's not very likely. So I'm savin' my money and investin' it. I figure I have only about five to ten good years at this. I'll keep up my workouts and my protein diet but the looks will begin to go; nothin' can stop that.

I know where I want to live: Tucson, Arizona. I spent a summer there and it's heaven to me: the open spaces, the dry air and sunshine, the mountains and desert, the friendly people. I hate it here in Boston and am only here because my family is on the Cape."

"But how will you earn a living in Tucson?"

"I've done a lot of thinking about that and some research. I'll open a coffee house with a big outdoor space in front. People will always want coffee and they like to sit with a cup and talk."

"You're very different from most escorts. They all have a fantasy but most do not have a definite plan on which they are working. Not at your age anyway."

"That is where I'm different from the others. They don't look ahead; they act as if what they're doing can go on forever and when they get to be thirty or so they're nothing."

"Your plan is very appealing to me; like you I love the Southwest. One thing I don't understand, though, and I may be wrong. You are a beautiful man and you have a beautiful future but you look unhappy. Why is that?"

Patrick jumped at so personal and accurate a reading; he thought only he knew this much about his inner life. "You're right. The thing is I'm a terrible worrier and I don't feel I'm making enough progress toward my goals. I exaggerate a bit about how much money I can make and so far I've saved very little. In fact I'm livin' from day to day but I own some nice things—clothes and video equipment."

Moved by Patrick's vulnerability and by his beauty I hugged him around the butt and thought how much I would like to see him attain what he wanted—by way of me. He felt the love in my embrace and snuggled in closer. We lay in a dreamy state for a time. I put my finger in my mouth to wet it and then gently made circles converging on his anus. He let that happen and when my finger tip massaged his sphincter he slightly lifted his ass as if to press for more. My fingertip dropped in but he knew that he caused the penetration and controlled its depth. When he pushed further the finger came to life and went straight in.

Patrick groaned ambiguously. Pain or pleasure? I bet on pleasure and gently massaged the inner surface. He groaned some more.

It must be remembered that this was more than seduction into acceptance of a new act. Patrick's sexuality was at stake. If he liked getting fucked he was to that extent gay. So I pursued the inquiry.

Very gently, almost imperceptibly, a second finger moved alongside the first. Nature has had the foresight to taper our fingers at the ends and so the anal sphincter is not at once outraged by some great knuckle and can relax its grip by degrees.

More groans from Patrick. If he were truly pained or deeply wounded in his *amour propre* he could, of course, throw me off. He did not. Therefore I took the groans to be saying: "This is not really me, but it's not bad."

After a while he said: "I can only pay attention to one or the other. I can't get off with your fingers up my can. So he turned over and with very little help and in very short order, climaxed. I concluded that he was incipiently anal and felt happy to have this gift to offer him.

* * *

Patrick lived in the South End, not in a single room but in a good-sized, old-fashioned apartment. His mate Mack was a commodities dealer, very ambitious, very handsome, very into brand-name cars and clothing and watches. And Mack was English, *very* English, Patrick liked to say. It was his Englishness, Patrick thought, that made Mack so very particular about possessions and manners and speech. Patrick rather idolized Mack and was grateful for his friendship, which annoyed me because I found Mack a familiar *type*, far from the best of that type that I had known, whereas Patrick was humble, handsome, warmhearted, and *original*.

Mack was straight and had a fiancée who was often at the apart-ment, too often for Patrick who unavailingly counseled Mack against marriage and indeed against women. Patrick could talk this way without anyone thinking him gay because he had been married and was so clearly what people think of as masculine. And Mack was so securely straight that he could say of Patrick's beautiful butt: "I sometimes think I'd like to roger him to death." ("Roger" is an English term for "bugger".)

One evening Mack and I did go to the Ramrod Club to see Pat-rick's show—the naked shower bath. It nearly killed Mack to find himself in the company of hundreds of obvious queens and he sought the seclusion of a rear banquette. Patrick came on at midnight with-out sufficient fanfare and in a faint and badly-aimed spotlight that resulted in his taking his make-believe shower with little attention from all the cruising, smoking, self-absorbed, half-naked little num-bers in the bar. I minded very much his failure to cause a stir, but Patrick did not. He went through the motions of a shower, taking on innocent pride in his magnificent body, but not looking lewd and not feeling lewd or really expecting to make onlookers feel lewd. To me there seemed nothing lubricious about it at all. He was a clean-minded boy showing what he had accomplished at the gym. It may have been all the real showers he took but there was just nothing "dirty" about Patrick. Nothing nearly "dirty" enough to make him a hit at the Ramrod.

Mack had to stand up on his banquette to catch a glimpse of the show and a glimpse was as much as he cared to have. With his head above everyone Mack became visible to the crowd and immediately attracted attention he found unwelcome. As we pushed our way out Mack said to me: "So what do you think, Roger? Is our Pat (his name for Patrick) going to end up as a homo or what?"

"Oh, I don't think so." How Patrick would "end up" sexually I did not know, but not as anything as simple as Mack's conception of a "homo."

* * *

Patrick had incredible social composure for one so young and seemingly vulnerable. It was Gregg Solomon who first found the name for the trait. Out of friendship for me Rebecca gave a small dinner party to introduce Patrick to a few of my best friends. Later he confided to me that he did not really enjoy it. That is no wonder, for as Gregg pointed out, he was really on the spot. Except for Patrick we all knew one another intimately, and except for Patrick we all had advanced degrees and were professionals, and he was certainly the only one who wore cowboy boots.

I cannot now imagine why I thought this dinner was a nice thing to do for him, but I did, and he did very well. Not in the way Skip would have, by advertising his naiveté and overcoming it with good cheer and boyish comedy. Patrick looked a little dour and judgmental and only spoke when he was sure of himself. He almost intimidated us, Gregg said, he was so composed.

I took Patrick to lunch at Biba's, an expensive and sophisticated restaurant. He asked for a California wine they did not have and raised an eyebrow at their provincialism. He returned my hospitality by taking me to a film at the Museum of Science. I had never been there and it was more thrilling than Cinerama and not expensive.

Harvard owns several properties on the north shore which it rents to faculty for a maximum period of one week in the summer at very reasonable cost. I had never taken advantage of this opportunity but, in the summer of 1993, looking for things to interest Patrick, I did. I rented for a week in August the William Dean Howells house in Wells, Maine. Jack, Skip, and I drove up in my car and Patrick arrived about an hour later in his.

The house looked wonderful at first. It was completely furnished and always clean because a regular staff spent a day polishing it between weekly rentals. It was on a height overlooking Wells Harbor which was always bobbing with colorful small boats. The Howells house was enormous, with five bedrooms on two floors. The dining room table was set for twelve. It was old and a little spooky which particularly charmed Patrick who gleefully imagined the four of us seated around that great table. What I noticed was that the house was also hot on that hot August day and you could not cool it because the windows were few and small and there was no air conditioning.

Jack, Skip, and I arrived in high spirits. The three of us had become a kind of family. We all liked one another and nobody lusted for anyone. I still found Skip attractive and always would, but he had long ago learned to manage me with lots of physical affection and real love but no sex. We could say just about anything to one another and did, and we laughed at the same things.

Into this happy family Patrick, at length, made his entry. Skip knew about Patrick and was not pleased about him as he had not been pleased about Grant. He wanted to have the first place in my heart, even though he was never willing to do the things that would certainly have procured it. And I was just as bad, envious always if Skip seemed to prefer anyone to me—which he often did. But now Patrick was first in my affection because, like Grant, he was willing to make love with me.

I remember Patrick's arrival—not as it was but as it felt. As it felt to me, guessing how it felt to Skip. It felt like a Hell's Angel had roared up on his motorcycle and swaggered into our sewing circle. In fact, of course, Patrick did not swagger but only walked without apology and drove a Honda, not a motorcycle. Still he was wearing very cool and opaque sun glasses and was about four inches taller than Skip who seemed almost to tremble.

Feeling the tension, Patrick suggested taking me—alone—for a ride in his new car. He knew very well how bad I felt for Skip and diverted me with remarkable success by stopping at a store devoted to "collectible" cards of sports stars, airplanes, and automobiles. I did not know that this store or this world even existed, but Patrick was a connoisseur able to ask learned questions about the prices and availabilities of cards that were evidently famous. I was the kind of intellectual to be immediately fascinated by a new domain with categories and structure nontechnical in nature. And Patrick accomplished what he intended: I lightened up and cooled down.

When we got back to the house, in less than an hour, Skip was gone—back home to Boston. He left behind for me a personally decorated box—left it as a gift but I felt it as a reproach.

I was in an agony of remorse until I was able to reach Skip at home by telephone and he assured me that he had just been sulky and felt better already. How many times the boy had made me suffer by reason of his deceit, and how many times he had enraged me, we know, but the love between us that began in this way was now such that neither could stand to hurt the other.

Jack and Patrick and I drove that evening into the nearby resort town of Ogunquit. Ogunquit was mainly gay in the 1950s and

1960s and Albert and I had often gone there with our friends Glen, Kevin, and Arthur. When that friendship ended Albert and I stopped going for about a decade. Then, one year in the 1980s we went back intending to stay at a guest house we used to like. The minute we stepped on the veranda it was clear that the "orientation" of the house had changed. The folk sitting there, with children and dominoes and card games, would have never have been there in "our day" and would not have looked away from us as from an unwelcome alien species. Clearly "our day" was over at that guest house, and as we soon learned, in all Ogunquit.

Patrick was the driver on the way back to the Howells House when a squad car pulled us over. "Shit! I was only doin' thirty miles per hour." But the limit on the road was twenty. Asked to show his driver's license it turned out that Patrick's had recently expired and then the police got rough.

"Face the car, hands in the air." They searched him, shoved him into the squad car and told Jack and me to follow them to the station. Inside the station they sat us on a bench and took Patrick inside for interrogation.

In the police encounter we saw more of the range of Patrick's composure. They threw him up against the car and searched him as if they thought he might be packing a gun. He remained calm though sullen and even put a trace of insolence into his replies.

Composure was certainly Patrick's leading trait but privacy was also strong. To grasp what Jack and I felt in the hour or so that we sat waiting the outcome of Patrick's interrogation you must realize how little we knew about Patrick. Jack said, not quite seriously: "For all we know he might be a baby-faced serial killer." I knew why we knew so little about Patrick. The second time we met he told me: "My dad always says play your cards close to your chest."

"Why should you do that?"

"So people won't know nothin' they can use against you."

Patrick turned out not to be a serial killer but only late in renewing his license.

Back at the house later that night I got into one of the huge beds with a little glass of vodka, and Jack and Patrick crawled in on either side of me. We all felt relaxed after the brush with the police and joked for a while. Patrick greatly enjoyed that nonsexual bonding time, he later told me. I fell asleep but Jack and Patrick went down on the porch and talked and drank most of the night. Patrick confided more to Jack than he ever had to me–mostly about his marriage to Mia. He loved her and missed what they had together and he cried quite a lot. Jack told me the whole story the next day and when I heard I wanted to leave as soon as possible.

I had been so foolish as to imagine that Patrick was getting seriously interested in me. In fact he said more than once: "I love you" and I was not in a mood to think about what he might mean by "love." But Jack, as often before, introduced a little reality into my wish-world, and it appeared on the evidence of their talk that Patrick was straight and pining for his lost love. Once I understood that, I could not get away fast enough, and since I had paid the rental we left after just the one day.

A few days later I received an anonymous note: "I understand that you are seeing a man who calls himself 'Patrick.' Let me warn you that he is a liar and a thief and you had best beware."

Coming on top of my general ignorance of Patrick's past and so soon after the encounter with the police, the note did disturb me. However, before telling Patrick about it I decided to trust him and not the note. The note sounded spiteful, and in any case everyone lies, and I had no possessions worth stealing except a huge, unmovable leather sofa.

When I told Patrick I saw him lose his cool for the first time: "That's Bill, that shithead. He runs the escort service and is pissed at me because I won't take calls any more. It's him that's the thief. He owes me fifty dollars. I'd like to beat the shit out of him but he's an old man."

The transformation was something to see. Who would have thought the boy had so much anger in him? I hoped never to be the object of that temper.

* * *

Jack and I had long planned to make a trip to Paris in August of 1993, and when he learned of it Skip started to work on me to take him along. He had a case. When I first fell in love with Skip I had the most capital I would ever have and the least interest in living except for Skip, who had, after all, pulled me out of depression. I am guilty of having dangled before him the pleasures of the world: what I thought of as wealth and also travel to Greece, Italy, Morocco, or wherever. The contingency was never spelled out but was, we both knew, complete and exclusive physical love. The poor boy went as far as he could but he just could not stomach it and then after all he fell in love, briefly but crucially, with in and lost his claim on all the dangled treasures. But not totally after all, since I had dangled and never quite said: "if you can bring yourself to love me." So when Skip said with reference to Paris: "I'm twenty-eight years old and never been out of the country," I felt some responsibility.

More consequential was the fact that I loved his company. Anything was more fun with Skip along and that would be true of Paris. So I thought I would like to take him, but now there was the alternative of Patrick. He was not high spirited and fun like Skip, but what did that matter; I was in love with Patrick. However, I took Skip, partly because I had not lost all sense of fairness. And while we were gone, Patrick moved to Miami.

For three weeks after our return I heard nothing from him and then he just called, very calm with no apologies or explanations.

"Well, well," I said.

"Well, well," he said.

"If you had taken me to Paris instead of Skip I wouldn't have moved."

"If I had dropped Skip at the last moment for you, what kind of person would I have been?"

"That's true. They think a lot of me down here."

"I'm not surprised."

"I've signed up to make a series of movies called *Sky Divers*. We've already made the first one; it's called *Diving Mates*. It only took three days to make and they paid me $1,000."

"That's good money. What kind of movies are they that only take three days to make?"

"They're gay porns. My picture is on the box, but my name is supposed to be 'Ken.' It's not great money; it's $1,000 for a 'pop' if you know what I mean. A few hours of unpleasant work, mostly waiting and retakes."

"Where are you living?"

"I'm sharin' an apartment with a gay porn star. You probably know

his name and may have seen him: 'Joey Davenport.' There's nothin'
between us. He's straight and so are most of the gay porn stars."

"I never knew that."

"Do you hate me for what I done?"

"Of course not; I love you."

"I still love you."

"Are you free to come up to Boston for a couple of days?"

"I'd do it." This was the answer I always got from Patrick. No
enthusiasm or even interest, just compliance or agreement as in
striking a contract, which is what it perhaps was to him.

I did not suggest that Patrick stay with me, but put him up at the
Cambridge Hyatt which was just a few blocks away. It had always
been my principle to provide separate quarters for any boy who was
my guest; so as not to force intimacy by proximity, I liked to think.
He and I would both have our privacy and independence, and whatever intimate contact occurred would be by free choice. In thinking
this way I was deceiving myself since the guest always felt some
obligation to provide intimate contact arising simply from the fact
that I made the invitation and paid the bills. It was absurd to think
that shared quarters would add anything to the felt obligation. What
the separation did do was give me a chance to be alone, to take my
bath and go to bed, without being constantly subject to probably
critical observation.

Skip had enjoyed the luxury of the Pierre in New York and Grant
the Ritz in Boston, but Patrick had to make do with the Cambridge
Hyatt because I had had more money at the start of these adventures
than I had at the end. Skip had wholeheartedly enjoyed the Pierre,
even knowing that it was only available for a short time. Grant
cared less about the Ritz and would have liked to plow the money
into his business. I would not permit it once we knew his HIV
status, and I came to care deeply about giving him a treat (whether
he wanted it or not). I offered the Ritz to Patrick, but he would not
tolerate the waste of money. Patrick cared a lot about money, and
thought he might enjoy a long-term gain by encouraging a little
frugality in me.

I mention this short visit only because Patrick said something to
me in the lobby of the Hyatt which registered permanently in
memory, verbatim and with perfect clarity, a premonitory flashbulb

comparable to Grant's "Thanks for dinner." In making the reservation for Patrick I had used a credit card to secure it against late arrival, but had neglected to say that all Patrick's charges for the period of his stay should be made against the card. In the lobby, after greeting, Patrick took me aside and, in cold flat tones I had not heard before, asked: "Who's payin' the hotel?" I was, of course, but Patrick was taking nothing for granted in what he clearly thought of as a business deal.

Soon after returning to Miami, Patrick broke his contract for the *Sky Divers* series because Travis, the producer, was a shithead who could not keep his hands to himself. Patrick also got a much better offer to make a movie in Los Angeles. The offer came from Merlin, the unchallenged top director of American gay porn. The "magician" as he was known in the industry, had only made eight films in eight years. The average director made more than that in one year. And the average director's films were withdrawn from rental in just a few weeks for lack of customer interest. All eight of Merlin's films were, quite incredibly, still in circulation, which is something like a textbook (e.g., Samuelson's *Economics*) staying in print for fifty years. Furthermore, scenes from Merlin's films were "anthologized on films with titles such as: *Magician I* and *Magician II*." He was the industry's one clear "classic."

It is curious that so limited a medium as gay porn could yield a "classic" as well as indefinitely numerous variations of quality short of "classic." The dimensions of variation are few. All important performers are young males, over eighteen and not much above thirty, and all must have at least a minimal "sex appeal." Of course the pool so defined is still very large.

There are more men than women looking for work today in X-rated movies and video. The Los Angeles suburbs in the San Fernando Valley swarm with men who have seen, on soft porn adult cable shows such as *Spice* and *Showtime*, men enough like themselves to put it into their heads that their physiques were marketable. Of the millions there are probably no more than thirty "stars" who can make a living. "Natural Born Killers" Faludi calls them in *The New Yorker* of February 30, 1995.

The repertoire of basic actions is limited to three: fellatio (cock sucking), fucking, and analingus (rimming). There is some small additional variation in terms of positions and number of participants. On so slender a pedestal gay porn produces annually something like 250 distinguishably different variations which can be rated for quality and have been since about 1970. The *Adam Gay Video Directory* has published five editions on a two-tiered system which accords up to five stars for overall video production, and up to three stars for sexual performance.

Individual consumers of gay porn make personal judgments which are roughly reflected in rental popularity. We do not know how much consensus there is on these judgments and know nothing about the structure of the distributions, but it would be extremely interesting to know these things and make comparisons with such distributions in fashion and art. Gay porn is probably less purely cultural than clothing and painting, and more heavily physiological. The editors of the 1995 *Adam Directory* write: "Three pluses are awarded to those few vendors that gave our panel of reviewers big boners for the duration of the production." Not a statement one easily imagines hearing from Yves Saint-Laurent or the director of the Museum of Modern Art.

When Merlin saw pictures of Patrick, he predicted, as any sensible man would, that the boy could become the superstar "bottom" of the business. Gay men sometimes identify themselves as "tops" or "bottoms" for obvious reasons. Such praise from Merlin naturally went to Patrick's head, and he signed up to star in a single film to be called *Huskies* for a fee of $5,000, and flew out to Los Angeles for several weeks' shooting. Merlin is a cripple confined to a wheelchair and so not the sexual nuisance Travis had been. From his wheelchair, however, Merlin has dreamed erotic dreams that have haunted gay men all over the world: two naked men in an otherwise empty, graffiti-lined subway car; two big studs, one in a leather mask, abusing a willing boy in a pool parlor; a three-way *seriatim* rimming in a smoky alley with motorcycles and leather vests.

Patrick thought Merlin was better than any of the competition because he worked more slowly and carefully, doing one film a year instead of half a dozen, but there is much more to it than that and most of it is, as with any extraordinary talent, unanalyzable. He knows that for gay men, peak sexual excitement goes with anonymity, male settings, dominance, risk of discovery, and a delicately calibrated approach-to-but-avoidance-of disgust. In his great scenes performers never recognize one another; they meet in masculine places like pool halls, in places that are public but secluded like alleys, and perform almost-disgusting personal services on command. There is never any sentiment aside from excitement, dominance, and submission; never any suggestion of continuing relationship. But all porn directors must implicitly know these things. They go wrong often in letting some action continue too long; the magician never does that. They go wrong in not being sordid enough or, less often, too sordid. In the end an analyst must just give up and say that the magician knows what gets gay men hot as few others do.

The artistic standing of all pornography, let alone gay male pornography, is extremely low, though in the early 1990s pornography has had a few champions (e.g., Camille Paglia), all female. Its moral standing is even lower, and many feminists suspect that pornography is an important cause of real-life rape and perversion. The reasons for the condemnation are pretty clear and lie deep in our history and culture. At the same time, there is clearly an enormous amount of hypocrisy. Practically all consumers of pornography are shamed faced about it but they are also very numerous. The same culture that condemns hard-core pornography approaches it in mainstream films and television. Oral and anal sex, for instance, have become commonplace in movies. Sexual language and innuendo are everywhere in the media. Our attitude is certainly two-faced and the moral and artistic cases against pornography have never been satisfactorily made. However it cannot be easy to see dignity in acting where "gettin' it hard" is the main achievement and "waitin' for work," as the stars of the medium say, consumes so much rehearsal time.

The official position, the politically correct position, is clear: pornography, especially gay male pornography, is beneath contempt. It is this clear official position that governed Patrick's next move: he would never make another pornography film. *Huskies* was it. Patrick's friend, Sean, had been in line for the cover of the magazine *GQ* (*Gentlemen's Quarterly*) but when the editorial staff discovered the fact that Sean had made a pornographic film the coverboy offer was withdrawn.

"Any pornography ever, and you are blackballed," said Patrick,

"So if I ever do have a career as a model or actor, porn would ruin it. I'm cuttin' my hair short and changin' the color a little and with the nose operation I'm gettin' I don't think anyone would ever recognize me as the star of either *Diving Mates* or *Huskies*." The nose operation was something he had long been saving for. He needed it to reduce a bad postnasal drip but it would also have a cosmetic effect. Modeling agencies had told Patrick that his face fell short of perfection only in that the nose was a little bit too broad. I, and others, believed that the idea of the perfect face was a snare and a delusion. One had only to look at male romantic leads in the movies to see that there are many types of facial appeal, though it is true that models show less variety. In any case, Patrick was quite right in thinking that no one would recognize the boy on the *Huskies* box in the All-American look he took on with short hair.

It is just as well that Patrick did not seek to become America's all-star "bottom" because *Huskies* turned out to be Merlin's first failure. The Adam 1995 *Periodical* gives it one star (the minimum) and calls it "definitely the weakest product" ever to come out of Merlin's studio. The *Directory* speaks of weak plot and errors of timing but I, as Patrick's close friend, have another theory—I think Merlin was defeated by the same thing that kept Patrick's show from being a hit at the Ramrod. He is a clean-minded boy, just not lewd or lascivious. Fucking is not his *fach*. I have never said this to Patrick nor shown him the *Adam Directory* review. He would think it a terrible artistic defeat.

When Patrick got his Miami offer and then his Los Angeles offer he just went, without phoning me or writing me until several weeks later. When he gave up pornography he moved back to Miami to wait for modeling agencies to hire him and earned his living as a hustler. I heard nothing from him and thought he had withdrawn from my life, but I missed him; not just for his looks but also for his impulsivity and crazy plans and sweet sense of humor. Patrick had got me past the grief of Grant's death partly because the two were in many ways alike: the same love of the Southwest, the same dream of a cowboy life, the same male arrogance and confused bisexuality. Like Grant, Patrick had brought some glamour into my life.

One evening in early October I was in my pajamas, reading. Thinking I heard a sound, I went to the head of the stairs and called down: "Who is it?" No answer. When my eyesight had dark-adapted I saw, standing in the darkest corner of the stairwell, in jeans and white shirt, Patrick! "What did I do?" he said.

"I forget," I said, still in the dark at the head of the stairs. Then I ran down and hugged him tight.

* * *

On February 1, 1994 I retired from teaching. Reluctantly, because the teaching I was doing was all enjoyable. Wonderfully talented undergraduates were coming to me for honors theses and winning *Summas* and Hoopes Prizes and Allport Prizes and Department of Psychology Prizes at an almost unprecedented rate. Doctoral students for whom I had major responsibility included Susan Field, Renée Oatway, Jasook Koo, Ronald Butzlaff, and Thaddeus Herzog—all of them by general criteria among the better students in the department. My two seminars were, respectively: "Social Psychology and Language," and "Masterpieces of Literature and Systematic Psychology." I limited the enrollment in each to just twenty and since each was always greatly oversubscribed, I could choose the membership according to criteria known only to myself, but talent was always the first consideration.

Japanese academics consider it very bad form to praise one's students since it is, after all, a way, very slightly indirect, of praising oneself—or bragging. They are right, of course, and in retirement one feels the lack of the support to self-esteem provided by gifted students. One also feels the lack of their gifts. The three young men I have loved since retirement—Skip, Grant, and Patrick—were as handsome as any Harvard students and in various ways as interesting. But they were not as smart academically or as well-educated. For all of them there were topics too abstract to be discussed, texts (like Shakespeare) too difficult to be understood. I always had to tailor my conversation to my conception of their abilities and they, no doubt, to their conception of mine. As Dodie said of Albert's brilliance, it makes such a difference. It is a difference like breaking into the stratosphere to go from conversation with any of "my boys" to conversation with my students; or Sharon; or Jack; or Rebecca; or Dodie; or a teacher-colleague.

In order to select students for a seminar I asked applicants to write a paragraph or so on why they wanted the course. "To fill a requirement" earned automatic exclusion. What really got to me was sly ingratiation. For instance: "I'm actually a chem. concentrator and I've spent three years filling requirements in order to get at the really good stuff like this seminar." It did not surprise me that this student later in the year authored the Hasty Pudding Show. I always kept the sex ratio even on the principle that a little sexual fizz helped sustain the intellectual fizz.

I had also a joint teaching assignment, with Professor Ellen Langer, "Advanced Social Psychology." Ellen and I are good friends, but very different in most ways. She is brilliant, beautiful, impulsive, assertive, and bubbles with high spirits. Me, you know. When students first heard that we would teach the course together they said: "Wow! They're totally different. What will happen?" We hoped our distinct good qualities would summate but the first time around, mutual subtraction occurred and produced a very dead class. After that, however, we found congenial roles and produced something like a chatty talk show. Ellen played herself–all creative and optimistic. I played the sage, critical and wise, to whom Ellen showed deference as well as rebellion. Typically Ellen would rattle on for five minutes and then turn to me and say: "Isn't that right, Professor?" It was fun and it was good too.

Ellen once asked me: "How come your students always break into applause at the end of a seminar? Mine never do that. What's the secret?"

"You have to feed them a final line that asks for applause. I sometimes say something about feeling it a great privilege to have had this class."

The last time I taught my fall term seminar (1993-94) I used a different line: "Professor Ellen Langer has asked me how it happens that my seminars always end with applause whereas hers do not, and I have admitted that I end with a line or two designed to milk applause. Now, class, as you know, Professor Langer's office is on this floor in the western corner and she is there now more or less listening to how this class ends. I suggest to you, if it does not offend your dignity, that you give Professor Langer a finale to remember.

The class was delighted to oblige; not only with thunderous applause but stomping of feet and shouts worthy of an opera house.

I told this little story at my retirement dinner in May. Ellen was master of ceremonies and about fifty students and colleagues past and present accepted the $150 a plate invitation, including many luminaries. The dinner was held–where else?–at the Boston Ritz Carlton. It must have been something of a problem to figure out how to honor me on retirement. A two-day symposium eventuating in a memorial volume is the highest compliment that can be paid but would not do for me because I have done seminal work in three fields–psycholinguistics, cognition, and social psychology–and these fields are worked by different people who would have little to say to one another if gathered together in a symposium. In addition, I had already been given a *Festschrift* (edited by Frank Kessel) on my sixtieth birthday, made up entirely of papers by my own doctoral students; so many of them have become famous in psychology that the *Festschrift* is a volume of rare excellence for the genre. The dinner at the Ritz was just right for me and I was greatly honored that so many were willing to attend.

I have worked in different areas because I like beginnings, times when the curve of new knowledge is rising steeply, when chunks of intellectual gold still lie on the surface to be discovered by whoever looks first. When the incremental curve levels off and new discoveries become hard to make, I tend to look elsewhere. This preference for beginnings is more than a professional one for me; it is a master trait. I like appetizers better than entrées, overtures better than operas, foreplay better than old in-and-out. The work I did most immediately prior to retirement was on politeness theory (the Brown, P. and Levinson version) and that is work entirely new to psychology and it would have been impossible to make up a roster for a symposium.

Most of the events in my life in Patrick's pornographic period were medical. I retired for medical reasons; the spinal stenosis had become so vexing that a wheelchair could not be far away. In the spring term I had two courses and I did not feel up to the walking, sitting, or even thinking that would need to be done. I would either have to submit to the risky back operation that Jack urged upon me or become a supine professor.

On the positive side I wanted to write this book. I had already written parts of it–Career Crisis, Face-Lift, Dream Boys, and Skippy–and I thought there was interesting new information here. Most generally about the idea (attacked in my 1986 *Social Psychology*) of evaluative consistency in personality, the idea that people who look good and act good are likely in all respects to be good and vice versa, not good. In my book I proposed instead that "Anything Goes" by which I meant that just about any trait, action, or appearance can be combined with any other in the same personality. My own recent life seemed to me to be a good example of the truth that "Anything Goes." Surely people who knew me only from reading me or being taught by me or working with me as a colleague would not guess the facts of Career Crisis, Face-Lift, and Dream Boys. In short, I was taken with the unexpectedness, the shock value of my personal life and wanted to disclose it as a contribution to psychology. I wanted to disclose it, but I also shrank from discussing it, and thought at the time of retirement that I might pass it all off as a novel. Later on I decided that it would be better to acknowledge it as an autobiographical memoir.

The theory of evaluative consistency has taken hard blows in modern times from candid tell-all biographies and from talk shows in which participants often do not look their parts. It is not dead, however, as we see every time a child molester or serial killer is described by astonished neighbors as seeming to have been a model citizen. And, as of March, 1995, all America was still puzzling over the possibility that O.J. Simpson, heroic in looks and most deeds, may have murdered two people. However I am less interested now than I was in providing evidence against the theory of evaluation consistency and more interested than I was in exploring the love lives of old professors in interaction with young male hustlers.

Jack told me there was a neurological surgeon at Massachusetts General who often relieved spinal stenosis and made an appointment for me. Jack always worked through the secretaries on my behalf and managed to convince them that his "uncle" (me) was a man of great importance in such dire straits that he must be seen sooner than the six months or so one usually had to wait. I walked for young Dr. Miracle both forwards and backwards, successfully touched my nose with my eyes closed and tried to stand on one leg

(I couldn't). He told me that stenosis sometimes improved spontaneously, but I told him that mine had been rapidly progressive for eighteen months, and for six weeks now I had used the cane he saw. He admitted that it could become crippling, which is what I feared. He had me get a myelogram to add to my stack of X rays and said he would be willing to try surgery.

"What will you do?"

"I actually don't quite know, and won't until I see inside your cord."

"What are the chances that surgery will make it worse? Might I become paralyzed?"

"I think there is almost no chance that you will get worse. Probably I can somewhat ameliorate your condition. That is the most we can hope for."

"You inspire confidence, did you know that?" (He smiled slightly.) "Let's do it."

We set a date for the operation, but well before that date I had one of my regular, every-six months, appointments with Dr. Hightower at Mass General who was in charge of my prostate. In charge really of its wake or aftermath since the organ itself had been removed five years earlier, even before Albert was diagnosed with lung cancer. The prostate had been malignant but "they got it all" as patients say and "no further treatment was required at that time" as doctors say. For prostate cancer there is a simple blood test: the PSA or prostate specific antibody. I always had this test just before seeing Dr. Hightower and for over four years now its value had been zero.

"You look very fit as always," said Dr. Hightower; an impressive man in a pin-striped suit, the best in the business, rumored to have removed President George Bush's prostate. "It's remarkable that you continue to look so well when you have had so much illness."

"A little suntan, doctor, should not be mistaken for health."

"Hmm. Well, I'm sorry to say that your PSA has, surprisingly, taken a small jump. It now reads 2.3. That is very low but we took it twice as a check on reliability. It means you have prostate cancer."

"Where?"

"We can't tell from the PSA; it just tells us somewhere in your body. With so low a number it is probably just at a biochemical level."

"How long have I got?"

"Oh, my dear sir, you have every prospect of being cured. We should begin radiation right away because our studies show that it makes a difference even at low PSA levels."

"How do you know where to radiate when you don't know where the cancer is?"

"We radiate the most likely site, which is the area formerly occupied by the prostate. You will need thirty treatments on a daily basis, five days a week. A treatment only takes a couple of minutes and it can begin at a time convenient to you, always the same."

"But I feel perfectly well except for the spinal stenosis. That is nearly crippling me."

"Prostate cancer is asymptomatic in the early stages, but if untreated it leads to bone cancer."

"I have a date for surgery on my spine in just two weeks. Can the radiation be interrupted?"

"No. You had better let the surgery wait."

"I don't think so; the crippling effects are too severe. The prostate isn't bothering me at all."

"Your stenosis will never kill you."

I went to the chief of urology at Beth Israel Hospital for his opinion. He told me that they would not radiate at all for a PSA level as low as mine and I learned that the two great hospitals took different "positions" on treatment for prostate cancer. "Positions" is the right word since the evidence on radiation and other therapies is ambiguous and so a hospital team (urologist, oncologist, et al.) must simply take a "stand," consistent within a team based on their view of the research evidence and clinical experience. Mass General, where I was being treated, judged that radiation at the earliest signs was the right thing to do. Nothing is known about the rising curve of the PSA—when it will be slow and when it will be rapid. The value "12" in Dr. Hightower's experience is the lowest at which he has known prostate cancer to become symptomatic. In October 1994, one of my colleagues, George Goethals, had a reading of "40" and was still free of symptoms, but in February 1995 George died.

I made a risky decision: to postpone the radiation and go ahead with the back operation as scheduled. If the back operation was successful I would make a short "dream trip"—sail on the Queen Elizabeth II to England because when I was young I had crossed the Atlantic by ship and loved the experience. I would spend four days in London staying at the Savoy Hotel—another happy memory. From London I would go to Rome and stay four days at the Excelsior which I know adjoined the Via Veneto—more memories. Then I would come back as fast as possible—which meant taking the Concorde in London, something I had always wanted to do. Promptly on my return I would start the course of radiation treatments which, by then, would have to number thirty-six. I did all that and lived, but the dream trip was no dream because I persuaded Patrick to go with me.

* * *

As I have said, Patrick stood in my hallway and asked: "What did I do?"

"I forget."

I ran down the stairs and hugged him hard. Sitting in the living room, I told Patrick about the dream trip but nothing about the medical stuff except that the back operation had been a success and I no longer needed a cane.

"Come with me. It would be so wonderful. Harry Ginger, my travel agent, can just duplicate everything, I'm sure. Another stateroom on the Q.E.II, a second room at the Savoy and at the Excelsior and another seat on the Concorde. And Harry is so good he can probably get us adjoining accommodations all the way."

"Let's think about it a couple of days."

"No, say 'yes' now. You're not doing anything special and this is the chance of a lifetime." I tried to capture his gaze. "Why can't you meet my eyes?"

"I don't know."

"How have you been living since you gave up porn films?"

"Hustlin'. I told you I'll never take a nine to five job for peanuts when I can make $300 an hour and not do nothin' much except take my clothes off. I tried the nine to five life when I left high school workin' as a construction worker. I don't mind hard work. I could show you half a dozen roofs in downtown Boston that I helped with, but they didn't pay shit. I couldn't even save up enough to buy a car. It just didn't make sense to me."

"But I thought you were doing well with your limousine service?" I had helped Patrick buy a secondhand limousine and he was doing well, I thought, driving the South Beach gay crowd. He told me he liked to tease the "boys" when they flirted with him by saying: "You couldn't afford me."

The night hours were not a problem for Patrick because he almost always stayed out until around 3 a.m. and slept the following day until well into the afternoon. What he did in his nocturnal hours before the limousine I never knew, but I believed what he told me: "Mostly people watchin' in clubs. Actually I feel very lonely in those crowds and people are always comin' up to me and askin' 'What's a good lookin' guy like you doin' all by yourself? I tell them I have a friend I care about—that's you—but he lives in Boston."

Jack and Skip thought I was crazy to believe this story, but I did and I do. With Patrick I had decided to be trusting and nonpossessive. There would not be anyone after him, I judged, and he was very lovable. So this would be my all-out try at finding a Primary Other.

"I sold the limousine. In the summer there was almost no business in Miami. And in the winter when it was busy it interfered too much with my life. If I wanted to come up to Boston to see you I couldn't because I had to look after the business."

"But when did you ever want to do that? You didn't tell me."

"Well, I thought of it. Anyway hustlin' pays better and the hours are better. Right now I hafta admit it's kinda slow."

"Well then, right now is a good time to take a vacation. Please say you'll come with me. I had the back operation partly so I could make the trip."

"In a way, then, you had it for me. Okay, I'll go. I'm gonna get a really good camera so I'll have pictures of us in Europe at least."

When Skip learned that I was taking Patrick he felt it as a deep betrayal. After all he and I had often talked of glamorous trips we might take together, and I had implied that there was no financial reason why we should not do so. One of Skip's favorite routines from the movies was: "How'm I doin'? Sal's takin' me to Italy—that's how I'm doin'." The accent is that of a Mafia gun moll. He took me home from the hospital after the back operation in the highest of spirits with balloons flying from the Geo Tracker. What might we not do now? No more teaching and me able to walk–a little wobbly and not far–but good enough. And then, first he heard I would take the dream trip alone because it would be so expensive. And now I was taking that sociopath, Patrick. To me Skip just said: "People do what they have to do, I guess" but Jack said Skip was very depressed the whole time we were gone.

As it happened there was little to envy. The trip was a sad affair. This was partly because Patrick and I thought of it very differently. To me it seemed that I was giving Patrick a marvelous treat and that is what it would have been for Skip. To Patrick it seemed that he was doing me–an old man and not strong–a tremendous favor. After all, he had to carry the bags and help me over the rough spots in the Roman ruins. Could I have made the trip at all without him?

After a week of truculence I guessed what was wrong with Patrick. "You are probably thinking of us as client and hustler! Would it help if I gave you $5,000.00 for your trouble?" It did. It helped a little but there was another problem not easily corrected. He was taking the trip of a lifetime with the wrong person. Not only was I not the dream companion, I was not even very good company for the twenty-four-year-old young man. He was an extreme nocturnal coming to life mostly at night, and I was an extreme diurnal, liveliest early in the day and asleep by eleven. Each of us kept to his pattern with the result that we did not have a great many hours of overlap. Fortunately the Q.E.II has gambling so there was something for Patrick to do after I went to bed. Each of us found something lovable in the other or we would never have made it.

One night in his room, clad only in a bathrobe, he gave himself a facial in the form of a green clay mask that you wash off after half an hour. In the green mask he looked like Jim Carrey in the film *The Mask* and he pranced around the room imitating Carrey saying: "Somebody stop me!" Then he let me in on his treasure trove of a dozen fine colognes. "Patrick, I think you can be the grandest courtesan in Miami or anywhere."

"Is that what you want for me?" I had not realized that he expected me to have a life plan for him and am still not sure he did.

The third day aboard ship at lunchtime I got tired of waiting for Patrick to wake up and went into his room, turned on a light, and said: "Lunch is being served." He always slept deeply, and in complete darkness, making a monkeyball with the bedclothes. "Turn out the light!" he shouted. I did and then stumbled and skinned one leg so badly as to have a permanent scar. He did not even look up.

The last night in Rome at dinnertime I sat at a desk eating one of the Excelsior's excellent pizzas when Patrick walked in jaybird naked. He knelt down about six feet away from me and slyly smiling, waved his erect penis back and forth. I tried to keep my attention on the pizza which was getting cold but, at a rapider rate, I was getting hot. I dropped the pizza and fell upon Patrick with my mouth full of tomato sauce. When he climaxed he looked as pleased with himself as if he had pitched a no-hitter–like the young man in the J/O show in San Francisco. More of an achievement than a pleasure.

The trip ended badly in customs inspection in New York City. We both had connecting flights to catch, different flights from different terminals, since Patrick was going to Miami and I was going to Boston. We would have had plenty of time to make our flights if things had gone smoothly. Our trouble began as we exited the Concorde. I hit my right hand against something or other, not a serious blow, very superficial, but the bleeding was profuse and persistent. I hopped along wrapping the hand in paper toweling and carrying my one bag in the left hand, urging Patrick to go on ahead since he had so much more luggage–four bags. I was making little progress when someone connected with the Concorde saw my plight and bandaged the bleeding hand. That slowed us up a bit, but the real disaster came with baggage inspection.

In one of the bars on the Q.E.II they sold beautifully shaped decanters with the ship's name on the outside and a fifth of fine Scotch on the inside. Patrick had to have this souvenir of his otherwise unrewarding trip. The decanter with the Scotch inside was so heavy I could barely lift it; Patrick easily could and bought one even though he had come against my advice with four pieces of luggage. He is a very strong man and he managed the lot with little trouble until we got to customs. The decanter was in a paper bag with handles and one could see the top but on the customs declarations Patrick had written that he was bringing in nothing of value from abroad. "And what do you call this?" asked the outraged inspector.

Noting a certain discrepancy of age and style the inspector had the impertinence to ask: "How do you two come to be traveling together?" I dearly wanted to say: "Unlikely as it may seem, we're lovers" but actually said: "Patrick is a former student of mine." The inspector found us an unsavory pair and so made us open every bag and account for everything within. Patrick snorted in outrage and that did not speed our progress. When the bags were finally passed, Patrick had only minutes to get to his terminal.

"Go! Go! For God's sake go! Call me when you get to Miami!" There was no time for proper farewells. I just sat down on the floor with a bag I could not possibly carry to the terminal from which the plane would leave. Indeed, after a long day of travel that had begun in Rome, I did not think my still-weak back would permit me to walk the distance. And what to my wondering eyes should appear but a college student–a black student from Boston with compassion in his eyes: "May I help you, sir?

He put me in a chair, the bag at my feet, and wheeled me to the plane. "Please write down your name and address for me" I groggily said, "so that I may thank you properly." I vaguely had in mind a four-year scholarship at Harvard but he just laughed and said: "My pleasure." There is a lot to be said for young men who are not hustlers.

I was home by 9 p.m. but poor Patrick was running to make connections and flying all night. He did not call till nearly noon the next day when he let me know that his return flight was one of the worst experiences in his life.

The trip might have ended everything between Patrick and me but it did not because I continued to woo him by letter and telephone. As the bad features of the trip faded, his affection–he would say love–revived. I think I have not made it clear what was lovable about Patrick aside from his body, but that is because I have not let him speak for himself. Here is Patrick in his own voice in a letter to me written on November 11, 1994.

Well this morning's phone conversation left me a little uncomfortable, I know you and your needs very well. I know when something is bothering you and when you're ok. What it is I think is you always need assurance that I can truly care for you very much. Well maybe you'll never know or understand but I do.

You're the first one I think of in the morning when I wake up and the last person before I go to sleep. I know that there are many miles between us and it can be as hard for me as for you.

I feel very upset that I won't be able to spend Thanksgiving day with you. Because you are in many ways more dear to me than my father ever was or ever could be. . . . I love you very much, Roger. I wouldn't change anything about you, everything that you are is what drew me close to you. I'll promise you that I will always be a part of your life in every way possible, you just need to trust me when I tell you this you are the dearest and most lovable person I have ever met. . . . You do everything in your power to make me happy, and for this you get my utmost love, attention, and respect and that also includes *trust*.

> Forever Yours
> Love Always
> Patrick

It is the letter of a very young man and Patrick usually did not live up to it in person, but it does warm the heart.

* * *

One Sunday Patrick called and he was crying.

"Honey, what's wrong?"

"Nothin'. I just feel so empty inside."

"Do you want me to come there?"

"No, no. I'll be all right. Probably I'm tired and I have a lot of stress. I'm scared I'll get AIDS like Grant did. I read an article and almost everyone who gets it is a gay man. And I'm worried I'll never be nothin'. My judgment is bad; I shouldn't have sold the limousine. And I don't have a circle of friends like everybody else does. I feel so alone."

"You're not alone; I love you. Do you want to see a doctor or maybe talk to Jack?"

"No, no. What good would that do?"

"Why don't you come up to Boston for a few days? I've been thinking about it, trying to pick a good time. *Angels in America* is opening here in a week. Have you heard about it?"

"People in L.A. were raving about it."

"I could get us tickets for Thursday on the same weekend that the Boston Lyric Opera is doing *Candide*. That's by Leonard Bernstein and I think you'd like it."

"I'd like to see another opera. The thing I enjoyed the most on our trip was *Cenerentola* at Covert Garden."

"You have good taste; it was an exquisite performance. The Boston Lyric is not up to that standard and neither is the Metropolitan most of the time, but the Lyric is good at finding young singers and since the house is small they can get a big effect. We can have dinner at Locke Ober which you enjoyed once before."

"I'd do that."

"Where do you want to stay? I'd love to have you stay with me but won't be offended if you'd rather stay at a hotel."

"Why don't I just stay with you."

"Great, you can have the larger bedroom and that way will have access to the TV and the front room."

"No, I want Al's room, the smaller bedroom. I'll be more comfortable there."

And so it was arranged and we did go to *Angels in America, Part I*. Patrick thought the second act was better than the first and third but did not much like it on the whole. It's about AIDS and Patrick got tired of listening to Louie whine. I did not much like the play either but that may have been because I found much of the dialogue, which is said to be very witty, unintelligible from our seats. When we got home about 11 p.m. I, as usual, got ready for bed. Patrick said:

"I'm goin' out and have some fun. In fact I think I'll get shitfaced."

I controlled my expression but felt cold horror inside, a horror fed by Skip's many dumpings at the Pierre in New York and by Grant's broken dates and behind all this forty years of feeling many evenings that Albert would rather be somewhere else doing something more exciting.

"You don't mind, do you?"

"I shouldn't, but to tell the truth I do."

"Why? This is your bedtime and I'm not goin' out to meet someone. I can't go to sleep at this time. I just hang out at the clubs. I won't really have more than a couple of drinks."

"I know, and I'm not suspicious of anything. I want you to enjoy yourself. But I do mind, Patrick, very much."

"You have to get over that. No one controls my life. I'm going. What's so terrible?"

"It's just that I could not do it to you, loving you, and so I can't understand how you can do it to me."

"I'm not doing anything to you; you're doing it to yourself."

And so Patrick went. I woke up at 3:30 and saw that he was not yet in. I woke again at 4 a.m. and he was blissfully asleep. I grabbed him around the neck and yelled: "Nothing is open in Boston after one o'clock. You've been with someone!"

He easily shook me off. "What's the matter with you? Since when are you an expert on closing times? There are a lot of after-hours bars, including the Loft, which is where I've been. Go to bed you crazy man! Don't you know I love you?"

And I did, saying: "You're right. I don't know what came over me."

Next day Patrick, Skip, and I were going to the movies together. We met in the apartment. This was the first time two of my "boys" had been together with me. Grant would never meet Skip: "There is nothing about him that interests me. Besides I don't like the way he treated you." Grant died soon after I met Patrick and so the two were never in the same place at the same time. Skip and Patrick had met—just barely—in Maine, but Skip had fled the scene. I often urged the two to get acquainted. They had so much in common and like-mindedness makes for friendship, doesn't it? Two other possible scenarios occurred to me: Skip and Patrick might be jealous of one another since both loved me; Skip and Patrick might suit one another so very well that they would tumble into bed together and then of course, I would have to kill them both. What actually happened was not a scenario I anticipated.

Skip and Patrick made common cause, generational cause, against me. Skip asked: "Has Roger ever 'flown into a rage' with you?" Patrick might have said: "Just last night" but he was too kind to humiliate me that much.

"Sure he has, but it doesn't bother me. I always remember the cartoon you drew. Remember? Roger in his pajamas sitting by the telephone which is not ringing at the expected time. And you show him tearing his hair out and a balloon from his mouth of exploding stars and pinwheels and fireworks. The memory of that cartoon always makes me laugh."

"The first time we were at the Pierre in New York he climbed on the window sill and threatened to jump."

"No wonder he likes opera; he's so operatic himself." And Skip and Patrick improvised an overwrought Italian operatic duet, striking all the poses with one hand to the chest and the other raised in the air. And collapsed in giggles.

I was developing one of my rages: "It's better than the idiot music you two play all the time: Country and Western and disco shit."

"Here's Roger when we were in London and Rome," said Patrick, and he bent over and hobbled slowly around the room and then espied a chair and speeded up, faster and faster as he got nearer the seat, finally collapsing into it.

"And how about sex? He's the horniest John I've ever met. It's all he thinks of."

"And the most inconsiderate. He always forgets to use lube. More lube, Rebecca, more lube."

The two were now overcome with laughter. Skip noticed that I was trembling with anger. "Are you okay?" He put his arm on my shoulders.

"Take your hands off me!"

"What's wrong? We're only kidding."

"I said, don't touch me. And I mean ever, you rotten little phony."

We went to the movie in order not to have to talk any more or see one another, and then we went our separate ways to our separate engagements. Two days later I wrote to Patrick.

Dear Patrick,

This letter will be essentially the same as a painful speech I just made to Skip on the phone. If I could be clear I would be, but I am not clear myself about why I got so angry when the three of us were together, but it has made a profound change in me.

It was the first time I came together with two of the boys I have loved. I should have been able to anticipate what happened since it is completely in accord with theoretical psychology, but I did not. Two people in agreement are a social consensus, and a social consensus defines social reality. The reality that came crashing in on me is that I am an old fool irrelevant to your young lives. So long as I was with one of you alone, and I always have been, I could overlook the reality in my absorption with the object of my affection.

What it means is that I have come to the end of a mode of adaptation to Albert's death and my retirement. Falling in love *seriatim* (one after the other) with three remarkable young men–Skip, Grant, and you–worked very well for me for three years. But now it is over, and about time; I am going to be seventy on April 14. I don't want to fall in love any more. I don't want to continue to misrepresent my tastes and convictions and knowledge in a vain effort to get close to someone young. I don't want the pain of comparing my appearance and capacities with the young. In short, I want to be with people my own age.

This does not mean that I do not love you and Skip and did not love Grant. It just means no more being in love, no more striving for sex and romance, and no more trips. I will continue to help you and Skip financially, paying the rents and car insurances and meeting emergencies. I am sure we will always be affectionate friends. What I most hope is that you both get the breaks in life that you have not had but for which you are so well qualified.

* * *

A week later Jack called: "Hello, Sweetpea. What are you doing for your birthday this year?"

"I'm going to spend it with Marian and Joan in San Francisco. I feel a need to be with them and they always want me and have for almost fifty years now. We can reminisce about Al together."

Chapter 8

Lie Down with Panthers

Following his conviction, Oscar Wilde wrote: "It was like feasting with panthers; the danger was half the excitement." I imagine his "panthers" to have been athletic feline young men with muscles rippling beneath velvet skin. And Oscar's panthers would have been working class. It was risky for a pale plumpish middle-class aesthete to lie down with such fellows, and they must often have unsheathed their claws and scratched him painfully. In the end they gave testimony that helped send him to Reading Gaol and into exile, but he never said that he regretted keeping company with them.

I was much older than Oscar and it was risky for me to pay to bring morally dubious panthers to my door. I was scratched many times until at the age of seventy I could take no more.

I spent my birthday with Marian and Joan. We did reminisce about Al and it was a healing time. Somehow, too, I knew it marked the end of this memoir. I had often wondered how I would know when the time had come to end. When you write a memoir that is also an ongoing record, you know that death can be counted on to do the job eventually, but you rather expect that, before death, things will come together, ambiguities will be resolved, and the meaning of it all will become clear. That never happened. What happened instead is that I realized I had stopped learning anything new. There was no satisfying closure in which everything obscure became clear and I attained enlightenment. The obscurity all remained and new ones were added but I saw that that was the way it would always be. The reason for ending the memoir at this point is that I think nothing new is going to happen. I have learned what I am positioned to learn about my subject—the love of old men and young—and that's it.

Odd that my curiosity should stop with an experimental sample of three because that happened to me once before, in my study of preschool language development in Adam, Eve, and Sarah. It was necessary then because transcribing the speech of even three children for two hours each week is very laborious work. Being in love with, first, Skip, then Grant, and then Patrick has not been laborious and it has not been research but it has taken a toll. It has involved my whole body and brain and heart. And quite a lot of the money I earned myself and the money Albert left me. He would be furious at this last "fine mess I have gotten us into" but I would not mind the fury if it meant seeing him once more.

Redundancy set in very early with Skip, Grant, and Patrick; even psycholinguistic redundancy which is the sort I am professionally equipped to recognize. Way back in January 1992 Skip wrote me the following:

> R,
>
> Your telephone privileges are hereby suspended [highlighted in yellow]. If you ever again leave a message like the last one I will have the number changed [highlighted in red]. I don't know what's going on inside your head but I don't want to see you until you get over it.
>
> S.

A little over a year later in February 1993 Grant wrote:

> Roger,
>
> I am hereby responding to the messages I received on my answering machine over the last two days. I feel sure they are indicative of your true feelings and have left a very sour taste in my mouth. Apparently you don't understand me at all. I cannot be owned, bought, or sold any easier than I can be told how to spend my time. I choose to do the things I do for very good reasons and resent being told by you that I am not at liberty to make such choices. If you don't have the ability to understand this then it is indeed best that we have nothing to do with each other.
>
> Grant

When I put these two letters side by side I thought I was losing my mind. In psycholinguistic tone they are identical. Both are brief and dispense with conventional salutations: no "Dear Roger" or "best personal regards." In tone, therefore, abrupt.

The first sentence of each is a performative. A performative is an utterance that accomplishes an act: "I hereby pronounce you man and wife" or "I hereby christen this ship the H.M.S. Pinafore." The word "hereby," which both authors use, is the very hallmark of a performative. Both were hereby revoking privileges and sundering relationships.

Performatives only work if what Speech Act theorists call their "felicity" conditions are satisfied. No one is wed when I pronounce them man and wife, and no ship is christened by my saying: "H.M.S. Pinafore." That is because the conditions that must be satisfied if the utterances are to accomplish their intended effects are not met. I am not authorized to marry people or christen ships, and essential persons and vessels are not even present. In short conditions are not "felicitous" (or happy) for the performance of weddings or christenings.

What are the felicity conditions for Skip to suspend my telephone privileges or Grant to end our intimacy? There aren't any that are substantial in nature since telephoning is open to all and so is friendship. However, there could be with a little escalation making a telephone number new and unlisted and declining to respond to a message. Both performatives are therefore still only threats but threats close to action. In any case they leave no question who is in charge; it is the author who threatens to act. It is clear what the threatened act would be: sundering an intimate relationship: ". . . don't want to see you," . . . "nothing to do with each other."

The final and most striking similarity is that both letters are written in what linguists call an "elevated register." An elevated or formal register in English is marked most clearly by the use of Latinate words of low frequency in preference to Germanic words of high frequency, *privileges* not *rights* and *suspend* not *halt* in Skip's letter; *respond* not *answer* and *receive* not *got* in Grant's. In such Southeast Asian languages as Japanese, Korean, and Javanese, elevated registers are much more elaborate and obligatory than they are in English and speakers are more aware of using them.

In all the languages we know about, elevated registers have two aspects. They acknowledge the high status of the addressee (e.g., a professor who is elderly) and, because elevated registers are more difficult than common registers, their use displays, or shows off, the linguistic expertise of the speakers–in this case Skip and Grant.

When I noticed these deep similarities in the two letters–similarities that make the letters almost the same act–I wondered if there was an Emily Post or Miss Manners handbook somewhere, *On Admonishing Presumptuous Elderly Admirers*. But I guessed not and thought the reason for the similarity lay in the social-psychological stance the two young men took to my anger and abuse: "I am in charge in this relationship, "both were saying," so you had best take care."

After all, in presuming to reprimand and even insult them in telephone messages, I had violated an understanding that it was in our mutual interest to maintain. This was no mere financial transaction, no simple exchange of money for youth and beauty, but a friendship, even love, on both sides. And so it was to be sure. We entered into it as equals, mutually attracted, and any suggestion of money or prostitution threatened our implicit contract. My telephone message broke the contract and their letters warned me that they were capable of blasting it apart.

Because money boys or hustlers (ugly terms that I hate to use) are selling what most people will not–access to their private parts and intimate services–it is important to them to be clear about what they will never sell but will preserve for merger with a self-chosen other person, a true love. There is always a sense of the inner self that is not for sale, that cannot be bought.

And so Karl Marx was wrong when he said he was an ugly man but also rich and with riches he could buy the most beautiful woman–and so was not really ugly at all. He could buy "services" as the homosexual John also can, but not love. He could buy compliance, as a social psychologist might say–compliance but not conversion. There is always an inviolable self, a heart of hearts that does not take orders. Shakespeare has Bertram say: "I do not love the lady and cannot strive to do it." The inviolable self wherever one may locate it is both a fact and a value. As a fact it is strikingly like the male erection—the one muscle we cannot flex. As a value it is the innermost treasure, the real self waiting to be won, not bought.

Skip and Grant and Patrick all were clear about this and sooner or later articulated it. One of the first things Patrick said to me was: "You can't buy feelin's." Later on, in outraged mood, he wrote: "I'm not changing for anyone. So you can accept me for who I am or you leave me the fuck alone. I don't need the shit." Skip after a serious session with a therapist said: "You can't buy me, you know." And Grant wrote: "I cannot be bought or sold any easier than I can be told how to spend my time."

And for many young men any approach to buying the self is stopped in its tracks. "I don't kiss" Because kissing one might slither up the tongue and into the heart. And often no direct eye contact—too close to the brain.

* * *

Almost every good-looking young man thinks of selling his looks. Not usually to men but to women, as porn stars. More men than women move to Los Angeles and try to break into the X-rated movie and video industries, millions more than the industries can employ. In this unusual business it is the women who are paid more—about 50 percent more than their male counterparts. They are more in demand. One man asked a female star for advice and she said dismissively: "Just get it hard" (Faludi, 1995). The men mostly come from sinking occupations: construction workers, bartenders, masons, mechanics. These are occupations in which you do something and they confer a certain artisan dignity. But they do not pay much. And a lot of men discover that nobody cares who builds something. Patrick used to be a construction worker. He worked hard and could point to a dozen tiled roofs around Boston that he had helped to build, but his name was not on any of them and he could not even afford to buy a car.

But Patrick is handsomer than 99.9 percent of construction workers, and people did care about what he looked like—both women and men cared—and would pay him well just for being and doing almost nothing at all. "What's the point in sweating your ass off for peanuts when you can sell your body for a fortune and not do nothin' you don't feel like? It doesn't make sense." That's the "Beauty

Trap" and Patrick was ripe for it, but in the end too smart to get caught by it.

The great majority of young men are not good-looking enough to fall into the trap but millions are, including many with college degrees who find they cannot find jobs that will even pay off their college loans. The Trap of Beauty, the reason why the gift can be fatal, is that it is sharply time-limited. Age inexorably deprives one of beauty. In ten years or so it is gone, and if your living is based on it you are nothing. Few things are so sad as the thirty-five-year-old hustler whose phone rings no more. There are not many of them, happily, because most realize that there is no place for veterans in the X-rated occupations.

For those who stay in the moneyboy business it becomes ever more important to preserve an inner self that is not in the business and will still be there—its beauty unimpaired—when at last, and soon, the whole man or woman gets out. Not infrequently there is a *real* boyfriend who does not know about the business, and for him the real feelings and also some affectionate acts are preserved. The terror is of being found out, and that is the end of everything real.

The irony is that, except for the truly dirty old man who is just that and nothing more (if such there be), the one thing he is hoping to buy is true feeling, the innermost self. It is a lonely universe, one of many it seems, and in passing through it one needs close company, a Primary Other. Grant once asked me what I wanted from him. His ass? I said that would be nice but it was really his soul I wanted. And what use would that be? I would be partnered by you in the infinite time ahead. And to Patrick I once said: "I can't expect you not to fool around. It's your heart I care about." And to Skip: "You're just a boy and highly sexed, but please let me know if you fall in love because that's what matters." And to Albert who once asked me why I wanted to hear a certain piece of music: "To hear it with you. Don't you know that sharing with you is what I care about?" In retrospect I wonder how we all came to be so wise. None of us were students of Plato's discussion of love and the soul, yet we had hit on the right terms concerning what it is the lover truly wants from his beloved.

The game of courtship between sugar daddy and moneyboy is not basically different from courtship in general. Surely what every true lover wants is the real self of the beloved. The difference is, I think, superficial if the courtship is extended in time as mine was with Skip and Grant and Patrick. The suitor offers whatever he has to give: gifts, charm, interest in the other's problems, attempts to share the tastes of the other, willingness to subordinate his own concerns to the concerns of the other. It is not too strong to say that he offers to give up his life for the beloved. The beloved cheerfully scoops up the material things offered and pretends to be, possibly is, close to giving up his heart's heart which is what the suitor yearns for. Probably the beloved cannot quite do it because we are here dealing with large differences of age and attractiveness and not thinking of Romeo and Juliet. Alas, all ye dear old men, Shakespeare probably got it right: "Whoe'er loves at all, who loves not at first sight?"

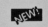
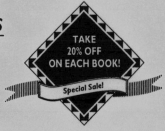